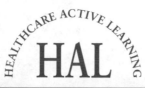

HEALTHCARE ACTIVE LEARNING

HAL

D0245886

EVALUATIVE
RESEARCH
METHODOLOGY
in nursing and healthcare

Start date

Target completion date

Tutor for this topic

Contact number

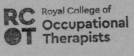

RC Royal College of
OT Occupational
Therapists

WITHDRAWN

USING THIS WORKBOOK

The workbook is divided into 'Sessions', covering specific subjects.

In the introduction to each learning pack there is a learner profile to help you assess your current knowledge of the subjects covered in each session.

Each session has clear learning objectives. They indicate what you will be able to achieve or learn by completing that session.

Each session has a summary to remind you of the key points of the subjects covered.

Each session contains text, diagrams and learning activities that relate to the stated objectives.

It is important to complete each activity, making your own notes and writing in answers in the space provided. **Remember this is your own workbook—you are allowed to write on it**.

Now try an example activity.

ACTIVITY

This activity shows you what happens when cells work without oxygen. This really is a physical activity, so please only try it if you are fully fit.

First, raise one arm straight up in the air above your head, and let the other hand rest by your side. Clench both fists tightly, and then open out your fingers wide. Repeat this at the rate of once or twice a second. Try to keep clenching both fists at the same rate. Keep going for about five minutes, and record what you observe.

Stop and rest for a minute. Then try again, with the opposite arm raised this time. Again, record your observations.

Suggested timings are given for each activity. These are only a guide. You may like to note how long it took you to complete this activity, as it may help in planning the time needed for working through the sessions.

Time taken on activity

Time management is important. While we recognise that people learn at different speeds, this pack is designed to take 20 study hours (your tutor will also advise you). You should allocate time during each week for study.

Take some time now to identify likely periods that you can set aside for study during the week.

Mon	Tues	Wed	Thurs	Fri	Sat	Sun
am						
pm						
eve						

At the end of the learning pack, there is a learning review to help you assess whether you have achieved the learning objectives.

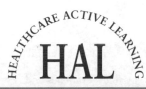

HEALTHCARE ACTIVE LEARNING

HAL

EVALUATIVE RESEARCH METHODOLOGY

in nursing and healthcare

Ros Carnwell

The Centre for Health Practice – Research and Development,
School of Health Science,
University of Wolverhampton, Walsall

THE OPEN LEARNING FOUNDATION

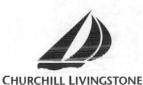

CHURCHILL LIVINGSTONE

NEW YORK EDINBURGH LONDON MADRID MELBOURNE SAN FRANCISCO AND TOKYO 1997

CHURCHILL LIVINGSTONE
Medical Division of Longman Group UK Limited

Distributed in the United States of America by Churchill
Livingstone Inc., 650 Avenue of the Americas, New York,
N.Y. 10011, and by associated companies, branches and
representatives throughout the world.

First published 1997

ISBN 0 443 057397

British Library of Cataloguing in Publication Data
A catalogue record for this book is available from the
British Library.

Library of Congress Cataloging in Publication Data
A catalogue record for this book is available from the
Library of Congress

Produced through Longman Malaysia, PP

For The Open Learning Foundation

Director of Programmes: Leslie Mapp
Series Editor: Peter Birchenall
Programmes Manager: Kathleen Farren
Production Manager: Steve Moulds

For Churchill Livingstone

Director (Nursing and Allied Health): Peter Shepherd
Project Controller: Derek Robertson
Project Manager: Valerie Burgess
Design Direction: Judith Wright
Sales Promotion Executive: Maria O' Connor

CONTENTS

OPEN LEARNING
FOUNDATION
TEAM MEMBERS

Writer: Ros Carnwell
The Centre for Health Practice - Research and Development
School of Health Science,
University of Wolverhampton, Walsall

Editor: Pip Hardy

Reviewers: Dr M Johnston
University of Manchester

Dr A Seed
University of Manchester

Series Editor: Peter Birchenall
OLF Programme Head,
Health and Nursing,
University of Humberside

THE OPEN LEARNING FOUNDATION

Higher education has grown considerably in recent years. As well as catering for more students, universities are facing the challenge of providing for an increasingly diverse student population. Students have a wider range of backgrounds and previous educational qualifications. There are greater numbers of mature students. There is a greater need for part-time courses and continuing education and professional development programmes.

The Open Learning Foundation helps over 20 member institutions meet this growing and diverse demand – through the production of high-quality teaching and learning materials, within a strategy of creating a framework for more flexible learning. It offers member institutions the capability to increase their range of teaching options and to cover subjects in greater breadth and depth.

It does not enrol its own students. Rather, The Open Learning Foundation, by developing and promoting the greater use of open and distance learning, enables universities and others in higher education to make study more accessible and cost-effective for individual students and for business through offering more choice and more flexible courses.

Formed in 1990, the Foundation's policy objectives are to:

- improve the quality of higher education and training

- increase the quantity of higher education and training

- raise the efficiency of higher education and training delivery.

In working to meet these objectives, The Open Learning Foundation develops new teaching and learning materials, encourages and facilitates more and better staff development, and promotes greater responsiveness to change within higher education institutions. The Foundation works in partnership with its members and other higher education bodies to develop new approaches to teaching and learning.

In developing new teaching and learning materials, the Foundation has:

- a track record of offering customers a swift and flexible response

- a national network of members able to provide local support and guidance

- the ability to draw on significant national expertise in producing and delivering open learning

- complete freedom to seek out the best writers, materials and resources to secure development.

Other titles in this series

INTRODUCTION

By the end of this unit of study you will be able to:

- describe the process of evaluative research
- explore the different areas within which evaluative research can be carried out
- specify types of research problems that would respond to evaluative research
- understand how data derived from evaluative research are analysed and presented
- design a small study using evaluative research
- explain the process through which the findings from your research could be disseminated.

Your knowledge of the research process as well as of methodology will be applied to evaluative research throughout the sessions in this unit. It is therefore essential that you approach this unit with a reasonable knowledge of both qualitative and quantitative methodologies, as well as of data analysis. **You should have studied the introductory unit and Units 1 and 2 of this series before embarking on this text.**

The unit is designed in six sessions, each of which contains learning activities. You may find that some of the activities take longer than the time suggested. This is perfectly acceptable, since the times allocated are only an estimate and it is assumed that some students will take longer than others.

Session One introduces evaluative research and defines the term, its origins and purpose. The session concludes with an explanation of the use of evaluative research in influencing policy formulation and decision making. This sets the scene for subsequent sessions.

Session Two carries the discussion of evaluative research further by recapping the qualitative and quantitative approaches to evaluative research covered in Units 1 and 2 and by discussing the value of inductive and deductive approaches to theory development using evaluative research. The session is designed to help you to select and justify appropriate data-collection methods to evaluate a programme.

Session Three explores design issues in evaluative research in more detail. We introduce the concept of formative and summative designs in evaluative research. Again, we draw on your knowledge gained in previous units in our discussion of experimental and quasi-experimental approaches to evaluative research.

Session Four explores a variety of approaches to evaluative research, each of which has had an appeal at different stages of the historical development of evaluation. This demonstrates how a change in emphasis moved the approach towards critical research methods. Five approaches to evaluative research are examined in this session:

- the experimental approach
- the goal-orientated approach
- the decision-focused approach
- the user-orientated approach
- the responsive approach.

Session Five draws on your previous knowledge of collecting and analysing data and applies this to evaluative research. The session takes you through the process of gaining access to relevant settings to collect data. You will then be assisted in selecting and justifying a sampling frame for data collection and designing questionnaires and interview schedules. Your knowledge of descriptive and inferential statistics will then prove useful in enabling you to analyse data from evaluative research. Finally, we will consider how to deal with qualitative data derived from open-ended responses and observations collected.

Session Six uses a number of articles reproduced in the *Resources Section* to assist you in reading and understanding evaluative research articles. The session concludes the survey of the research process by considering how findings from evaluative/critical research can be used to influence decision making. The session will assist you in planning strategies to disseminate findings from evaluative research in order to influence service delivery. Methods of communicating your findings are discussed, including giving final reports, articles for journals and verbal presentations at conferences.

LEARNING PROFILE

Below is a list of anticipated learning outcomes for each session in this unit. You can use it to assess your current level of knowledge and identify key areas on which you particularly need to focus. The learning profile is not intended to cover all the points discussed in each session, but provides a framework for you to decide how the unit can help you develop a fuller understanding of evaluative research methodology.

For each of the learning outcomes listed below, tick the box that corresponds most closely to the point you feel you are at now. This will provide you with an assessment of your knowledge, understanding and confidence in the areas that you will study in this unit. There is a similar exercise to complete at the end of the unit to help you review what you have learned.

	Not at all	Partly	Quite well	Very well

Session One

I can:

- define evaluative research ☐ ☐ ☐ ☐

- outline the purpose of evaluative research ☐ ☐ ☐ ☐

- distinguish between evaluative research and exploratory research ☐ ☐ ☐ ☐

- explain the use of evaluative research as an example of critical research methodology ☐ ☐ ☐ ☐

- discuss how evaluative research can be used to influence policy formation and decision making. ☐ ☐ ☐ ☐

	Not at all	Partly	Quite well	Very well

Session Two

I can:

- recall the meaning of qualitative and quantitative research

☐	☐	☐	☐

- describe the 'black box' and give examples of the methods of data collection used for each approach to evaluative research

☐	☐	☐	☐

- explain inductive and deductive approaches to theory development in evaluative research

☐	☐	☐	☐

- define the meaning of triangulation as it applies to evaluative research.

☐	☐	☐	☐

Session Three

I can:

- distinguish between formative and summative designs in evaluative research

☐	☐	☐	☐

- distinguish between experimental and quasi-experimental design in evaluative research

☐	☐	☐	☐

- understand the notations used in experimental and quasi-experimental designs

☐	☐	☐	☐

- explain how to design an evaluative research study to establish the value of a programme.

☐	☐	☐	☐

Session Four

I can:

- describe the advantages and disadvantages of the following approaches to evaluative research:

	Not at all	Partly	Quite well	Very well
experimental	☐	☐	☐	☐
goal-orientated	☐	☐	☐	☐
decision-focused	☐	☐	☐	☐
user orientated	☐	☐	☐	☐
responsive	☐	☐	☐	☐

	Not at all	Partly	Quite well	Very well

Session Four *continued*

- describe why the responsive approach is an example of critical research methodology.

| | ☐ | ☐ | ☐ | ☐ |

Session Five

I can:

- plan how to gain access to relevant settings for data collection purposes

| | ☐ | ☐ | ☐ | ☐ |

- select and justify a choice of sampling frame for data collection

| | ☐ | ☐ | ☐ | ☐ |

- design questionnaires and interview schedules appropriately

| | ☐ | ☐ | ☐ | ☐ |

- use descriptive and inferential statistics to analyse survey data from evaluative research

| | ☐ | ☐ | ☐ | ☐ |

- recall how to use qualitative data analysis to analyse open-ended responses and observations derived from evaluative research.

| | ☐ | ☐ | ☐ | ☐ |

Session Six

I can:

- understand research-based articles in the field of evaluative research

| | ☐ | ☐ | ☐ | ☐ |

- plan strategies to disseminate research findings and influence service delivery

| | ☐ | ☐ | ☐ | ☐ |

- prepare findings from evaluative research as:

a written report

| | ☐ | ☐ | ☐ | ☐ |

a journal article

| | ☐ | ☐ | ☐ | ☐ |

a conference paper.

| | ☐ | ☐ | ☐ | ☐ |

An introduction to evaluative research

Introduction

Evaluative research is a particularly useful approach to research in health and social care because it enables us to determine the value of the services we provide. We will begin by defining evaluative research and then discuss its purpose in relation to health and social care. We will distinguish between evaluative research and exploratory research and go on to explore how some types of evaluative research could be described as critical research. The session concludes by looking at the use of evaluative research in influencing policy formulation and decision-making – and thus sets the scene for subsequent sessions.

Session objectives

When you have completed this session you should be able to:

- define evaluative research

- outline the purpose of evaluative research

- distinguish between evaluative research and exploratory research

- explain the use of evaluative research as an example of critical research methodology

- discuss how evaluative research can be used to influence policy formulation and decision-making.

1: What is evaluative research?

Evaluative research is an approach to research which seeks to establish the value of a programme (or service) to the recipients. Programmes could include any health or social service provision. Packages of care for older people could be described as a 'programme' deserving evaluation, for example. Equally, a health education campaign aimed at a group of school children, or a series of parenting classes could be described as programmes. In fact, every time you set out to measure the effectiveness of the service you are providing you are engaged in 'programme evaluation'.

It is important at the outset to distinguish between evaluative research and exploratory research. This distinction is important because both evaluative research and exploratory research are used frequently in researching health and social care. The main difference between these two types of research is that, while evaluative research is used to measure the effectiveness of existing or developing services, exploratory research literally 'explores' a particular aspect of health or social care with a view to finding out how participants feel about it. The following two case studies illustrate the difference between these two approaches.

Evaluative research

Sally is a nurse working in an out-patient department. The department has recently introduced a new appointment system to reduce the time people have to wait after arriving for their appointment with a consultant. Sally has been asked by her manager to find out how effective this new system has been.

Sally evaluates the new system by documenting the time of arrival of each patient into the department. She also finds out from each patient the time of his or her appointment because some patients arrive before their appointment is due. She then documents the time that each patient is called in to see the consultant. This information enables Sally to calculate how quickly each patient is seen after entering the department. Sally can use this information to compare waiting times since the introduction of the new system with the waiting times before the system was introduced. If waiting times have reduced, Sally may conclude that the new system is effective.

Exploratory research

Ruth is a district nurse who specialises in the care of terminally ill people (palliative care). She is interested in finding out about the needs of relatives following the death of terminally ill patients. Ruth therefore interviews bereaved relatives over a six-month period. The interview also serves as a counselling session, so that she is carrying out her duties at the same time as collecting the data.

When Ruth finds out what the needs of bereaved relatives are, she can then plan her services to meet these needs.

As we can see from the first case study, the purpose of evaluative research is to determine whether any changes need to be made to a service or, indeed, whether it is so ineffective that it should be withdrawn. This can be quite threatening to the people providing the service (Polit and Hungler, 1987). As Popham (1993) points out, people don't like to be evaluated because they may be found wanting. This, he says, includes health educators who do not wish to expose their health education programmes to scrutiny. In order to gain the co-operation of their participants, evaluative researchers therefore need to add diplomacy to their research skills. Polit and Hungler also suggest that staff may be uncooperative because they are so convinced that their programme is good that they don't wish to waste valuable time, normally spent on caring, in assisting a researcher.

The second case study shows that the purpose of **exploratory research** is to find out more about the needs of particular clients or patients, so that future services can be planned to meet their needs. This is less threatening to staff because their performance is not being judged. Exploratory research takes place before services are developed, whereas evaluative research takes place either during or after service development.

Exploratory research: *An approach in which the researcher explores the field of research in order to seek the opinions and feelings of the participants.*

ACTIVITY 1 — ALLOW **10** MINUTES

Think about your recent working practices.

1 Give examples of occasions when you have evaluated programmes of care.

2 Give examples of practices in which you are currently involved that could be described as programmes and which are worthy of evaluation.

Commentary

1 There are many examples of programme evaluation in which health and social care workers are likely to become involved. The introductory unit of this programme introduced a range of research possibilities for health and social care workers, some of which could be described as evaluative research – for example, the evaluation of the transfer of people with learning disabilities from hospital to community settings and an evaluation of services for older people since the implementation of community care policies. We also discussed the use of evaluative research in measuring the effectiveness of this learning package in helping you to achieve your learning goals.

2 Many research problems are worthy of exploration but do not actually result in measuring the effectiveness of a particular service or programme. Two examples of research questions worthy of exploration, but which could not result in measuring the effectiveness of a service provision are:

- what is the experience of fathers who are present during the birth of their children?

- what are the supervision needs of social workers when first qualified?

The findings of the studies for both of these could influence the provision of services. However, in their present form neither is an example of evaluative research because a new service is not being established. The two examples could be reformulated as evaluative research in this way:

- how satisfied are new fathers with the support they receive during the birth of their babies?

- how effective is the supervision given to newly qualified social workers?

Two factors differentiate the two sets of questions above.

- The first two questions are exploratory because they are finding out about peoples' experiences and needs, rather than assuming that a service is already in operation.

- The second two questions assume that a service is already in operation and that its effectiveness can be measured. Note that there are key words in both of the last two questions which indicate that effectiveness is being measured – 'satisfied' in the first question and 'effective' in the second.

ACTIVITY 2　　　ALLOW 20 MINUTES

Below is a list of research questions or problems. Tick the boxes to indicate whether or not you think these questions are amenable to evaluative research.

	Amenable to evaluative research	Not amenable to evaluative research
1 What factors influence a woman's decision to breast- or bottle-feed?	☐	☐
2 Will the incidence of sudden infant death syndrome (SIDS) reduce if babies sleep on their backs?	☐	☐
3 How satisfied are travelling families with the care they receive from health professionals?	☐	☐
4 How effective is the triage system (a method of allocating waiting times to patients according to the severity of their condition) as a method of responding to patients' needs in an accident and emergency department?	☐	☐

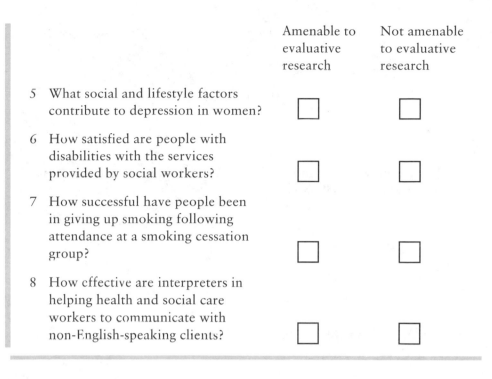

	Amenable to evaluative research	Not amenable to evaluative research
5 What social and lifestyle factors contribute to depression in women?	☐	☐
6 How satisfied are people with disabilities with the services provided by social workers?	☐	☐
7 How successful have people been in giving up smoking following attendance at a smoking cessation group?	☐	☐
8 How effective are interpreters in helping health and social care workers to communicate with non-English-speaking clients?	☐	☐

Commentary

You will find that the questions using an evaluative research approach all have something in common. They all make reference to some quality indicator such as 'satisfaction', 'effectiveness' or 'success'. Look again at the list and see which words indicate quality. Then see if these questions are those you identified as amenable to evaluative research. Questions 3, 4, 6, 7 and 8 all make reference to effectiveness, success or satisfaction. It is by measuring these factors that we can achieve some indication of how valuable a programme is. You probably also noted that these five questions assume that some programme or service is being provided and that the researcher is attempting to measure the users' perceptions of its success.

So what about the other three questions 1, 2 and 5? In their present form these questions are not amenable to evaluative research, but are good examples of exploratory research. Clearly it helps if we can find out about the needs and characteristics of people *before* we plan our services, and exploratory research findings may help us to do this. In relation to question 1, for example, midwives might benefit from finding out what factors influence a woman's decision to breast-feed so that they can deliver their health education messages more effectively. Discussing the convenience of breast-feeding may have little impact if the main factor discouraging mothers from breast-feeding is their embarrassment at the female breast being a secondary sex organ. Question 2 concerning SIDS is arguably closer to evaluative research, although it is not phrased appropriately for use in this way – in its present state there is no actual service provision to evaluate. Question 5 enables us to find out more about a group of people who are badly in need of mental health services. Once we have used exploratory research to identify their needs it would be very useful to plan programmes of care for this group which can subsequently be evaluated.

ACTIVITY 3   ALLOW 20 MINUTES

Look below at the three questions from the last activity that we decided were not amenable to evaluative research. Now change the focus of the questions so that they *are* amenable to evaluative research, rather than being exploratory.

1   What factors influence a woman's decision to breast- or bottle-feed?

2   Will the incidence of sudden infant death syndrome (SIDS) reduce if babies sleep on their backs?

3   What social and life style factors contribute to depression in women?

Commentary

Examples of how these questions could be re-focused are:

1   How *effective* are midwives in influencing a woman's decision to breast-feed?

2   How *successful* is a parental education campaign which was introduced in order to reduce the incidence of SIDS?

3   How *effective* are community psychiatric nurses in enabling depressed women to understand the factors contributing to their condition?

We have seen that, in designing a research question amenable to evaluative research, we are concerned with quality indicators such as effectiveness, success and satisfaction which can be measured. You may have noticed that in using quality indicators we are often measuring the effectiveness of services provided by specific professional groups or bodies, such as midwives or community psychiatric nurses. If any aspect of these services is found to be ineffective, then changes may need to be made to make them more beneficial to clients.

Interestingly, the use of evaluative research to improve service provision for users often places the researcher in the position of client advocate. The researcher may, for example, discuss with a community group the methods they can use to gain access to scarce resources and the researcher might then want to argue the clients' case to the relevant bodies. When the researcher takes on this role this research can be described as **critical research**. We will now go on to look at how evaluative research, in which the researcher gets involved with participants in order to instigate political change, can be described as critical research methodology, but before doing so we need to consider what exactly is meant by critical research methodology.

Critical research:
A research approach in which the researcher gets involved with participants in order to enable and empower them to instigate social and political change.

2: Critical research methodology

In most types of research, the researcher is mainly concerned with collecting data (both qualitative and quantitative) to explore and describe the nature of service provision, or to evaluate its effectiveness. However, clients' lives may be improved as a result of the research only if service providers are willing and able to respond in an appropriate manner to the researcher's findings. In this situation, however, the researcher is passive in terms of instigating change.

Critical research is a qualitative type of research in which the researcher actually gets involved in the lives of the participants in order to make life better for them. The critical researcher uses only qualitative methods, because it is these which enable him or her to become close enough to clients to help them to bring about social change. Here, the researcher is more active in instigating change and therefore may become a political activist. For example, the researcher could use the research process to help the participants to gain access to scarce resources by lobbying local government to demand extra pre-school provision for local children. The researcher could either act as an advocate on behalf of the client, or could empower clients by passing on their knowledge to the clients so that they have the confidence to act on their own behalf. Critical researchers often favour the latter approach because it enables clients to become emancipated.

As a health and social care researcher you are probably interested in making life better for the participants of your research – indeed this is probably the reason why you entered your chosen profession. Improving life for your participants may require that you understand their world and all the difficulties they face in their daily life. Understanding others' experience may be one of the aims of your research and may include an understanding of how people gain access to health and social services. Is access equal to all? Do people with higher incomes and living in certain areas have a better access than other, less fortunate people? Your research findings may be influenced by social factors (social class), culture (ethnic grouping) or politics (local political decisions determining resources). Once the evaluative researcher starts asking questions about equality and access in analysing the value of service provision he or she is using critical research.

One word that sums up the interest of the critical researcher, then, is 'equality', for critical research is concerned that participants have equal access to resources regardless of age, race, gender, disability or sexual orientation. Critical research is at the opposite end of the continuum to **positivism** – the belief that truth can only be found using quantitative methods with large sample sizes and tight control over experiments.

Positivism: *An approach to research which relies on the search for objective truth through quantitative measurements.*

Do we therefore need to abandon positivism altogether in health and social care research? Although positivism has limitations, the answer has to be no. If it had not been for positivist enquiry heart transplants would not have been developed, and we would not have access to such a wide range of antibiotics. These are just two examples of advances in medical technology which relied on laboratory experiments, i.e. positivist methods. In the same way, the positivist approach of using surveys of large samples of populations has also shown the extent and distribution of certain diseases so that resources can be distributed where they are most needed.

Research examples of critical research methodology

The following case studies show applications of critical research methodology to research.

Sakbinda is a health visitor working in a busy urban area. In addition to a large case load she is responsible for the health of residents on a large site for travelling families. The site is the only one in the city and Sakbinda wishes to evaluate the access to health services of the residents. She uses a critical research methodology approach by carrying out a study to assess the health needs of the travelling population in the area, as well as the developmental needs of their children and the effectiveness of local services in meeting these needs. After seeking permission to carry out the study, she carries out in-depth interviews of each family group. She focuses the interviews on health and development needs to ensure that participants don't divert the discussion to social needs. She discovers the following problems:

- families rarely use health services because they are inaccessible

- very few of the children have been immunised because parents don't think it is necessary

- facilities for disposal of waste and refuse are inadequate

- attendance of children at school or pre-school provision is spasmodic due to lack of acceptance by the local community.

Having discovered the health needs of travelling families, Sakbinda has two choices. She can either:

- act on behalf of (as an advocate for) the travelling families by informing service providers what services need to be provided, or

- work with the families, informing them of the procedures they need to follow to gain access to scarce resources and of ways they can inform decision makers about travelling families' needs .

Joe is a social worker who is particularly concerned with services for homeless people. He works in an area of deprivation in which bed and breakfast accommodation is frequently used to house families with young children. He is particularly concerned about the welfare and protection of young children in this type of accommodation and wants to find out how satisfied people are with the welfare services provided. He uses a critical research methodology approach by setting up a small discussion group for parents in bed and breakfast accommodation. Through group discussions he is able to discover what type of support is needed for these families. He discovers in particular that they need:

- crèche facilities for the children
- parent support groups
- help with budgeting and with completing benefit application forms applying for benefits
- help with developing skills needed to seek employment.

Having discovered what participants feel they want, Joe can then work with them to instigate the development of the facilities they need. Like Sakbinda, he can either act on behalf of the families or help them to seek the support they need to set up their own groups and meet their own needs. The parent support group, for example, could be set up by the families with Joe's help. This process of helping people to set up their own facilities is often referred to as 'empowerment' and it is often through this process that people achieve more control over their circumstances and become 'emancipated'.

In the first case, Sakbinda could empower the travelling families to seek their own solutions to their problems by discussing how to gain access to resources. Once the families have access to the same information that Sakbinda has, they can become more powerful in stating what their needs are. As a health or social worker you may have found that you have access to information that enables you as an individual to gain access to resources that you need. If, for example, you were unhappy with a hospital consultant you had an appointment with, you would probably have the confidence and the knowledge needed to ask your general practitioner (GP) for an appointment with a different consultant who might be more helpful. People who have knowledge are powerful. By sharing this knowledge with less powerful people you enable them to gain some power for themselves and thus give them the confidence needed to state their needs.

Emancipation often occurs as a result of empowerment. When you share your professional power with less powerful people they become more confident. If they become sufficiently confident to develop their own services they can become 'liberated'. If Joe helps a group of people in bed and breakfast accommodation to set up a parent support group he will at first probably be quite active in instigating this because of his professional expertise. However, once the group is running, natural leaders will emerge and they may take over some of the responsibility from Joe. This can be liberating for participants, who may move from feeling constrained by professional input to feeling free to manage their own lives.

These two concepts move the emphasis of the research from the researcher to the participants. Thus we can see that the researcher can have a dual role: not only can he or she act on behalf of the participant as an advocate and activist, but he or she will also facilitate the emancipation of the participants by empowering them to become activists themselves. The information collected from research will be used, not only by the researcher, but also by the participants themselves, in order to demonstrate to policy-makers the need for change.

The critical research approach illustrates that there is probably little point in evaluating the services you provide if the opportunity to effect change is not available. Critical research also illustrates the link between programme evaluation and decision-making. Since decision-making is often linked with local politics, evaluative research is often more overtly political than other approaches to research.

The evaluative researcher will not always be in a position to effect change. For example, the researcher could be restricted to improving a programme for the benefit of administrative staff rather than the participants. Here, decision-makers might insist that administrators, rather than users, were interviewed about their views concerning the length of waiting times for patients following the installation of a new computer system. Obviously this could not be described as critical research. However, as part of the evaluation process, a researcher can work with participants to develop strategies in which the participants themselves can *demand* an improvement in the programme. The earlier case study showed how a health visitor could work with travelling families to help them to demand resources.

If you decide to use a critical research approach to evaluation you need to be aware that your role as a political activist may cause conflict between you and decision-makers. For example, if you were evaluating the services provided by an elderly person's home and a group of residents told you that some members of staff deny them access to certain privileges, this might raise issues about the selection and training of staff which could prove costly to decision-makers. Because residents are vulnerable and not always in a position to defend their positions, you could act on their behalf by confronting decision-makers with the research findings. This could create conflict. You might indeed experience a personal conflict yourself between the desire to evaluate the programme on behalf of the decision-makers and the desire to act on behalf of participants to ensure that they get an adequate service.

Acting on behalf of participants in this way places you in the position of 'advocate' and 'activist' and moves the methodology of critical research well beyond the simple collection of data to facilitate change. Evaluative research can point out the strengths and weaknesses of existing programmes or services: Greene (1994) states that this information may influence resource allocation and power.

The following case study offers an example of the way information gained from evaluative research can be used to influence the allocation of resources.

Hospital trust: A hospital that provides contracted health services within quality and quantity specifications to a number of purchasers for an agreed fee.

Mary is a manager for a **hospital trust** and part of her job is to manage the hospital budget. This is an important position and part of her salary is performance related. This means that she must spend money wisely, be efficient and ensure that adequate services are provided in return for her salary.

Being a budget-holder is not an easy task. Mary needs to make decisions about spending money on potentially life-saving equipment and since she is unlikely to have sufficient money to purchase all the necessary equipment, priorities will have to be made. Does she respond to the need for innovative equipment in the Physiotherapy Department, new X-ray equipment to replace worn-out machinery in the Radiology Department or for an additional renal dialysis machine? Here she has problems associated with making decisions about whether to:

● buy new innovations (which may be more effective)

● replace old essential equipment

● buy additional essential equipment.

If Mary responded to the needs of all three departments she would probably run out of money quite quickly. Also, there may be many other resources required throughout the hospital about which she is unaware.

There are, of course, other areas to consider besides the purchase of equipment. For example, Mary needs to decide what proportion of the budget should be allocated to staffing, including types and grades of staff, and what proportion should be allocated to equipment. She will also have to consider the need for new buildings and whether to close wards.

In an ideal world Mary would not need to prioritise and would only consider the needs of patients. If new equipment was needed she would purchase it because it would benefit patient care and if the money ran out more would be found. However, nowadays managers work with strict budgets, and in order to gain an impression of the relative budgetary requirements, Mary will have to start by seeking the views of staff. As stated above, staff have competing needs and Mary may not have the funds to respond to all of them. She may decide, therefore, not to consider the views of individual members of staff about what equipment to purchase, but simply to talk to administrators. Administrators would be responsible for auditing the amount allocated to different items, such as syringes, and for determining how many are used each month. They would also have information about the different types of staff and how much they are paid.

Major decisions, such as building new departments or closing wards and departments, are made by a group of very senior managers and Mary would also need to seek their advice in relation to capital expenditure. In addition, local pressure groups may seek to influence the decision-making process by campaigning against ward closures or demanding that money is spent on certain equipment.

Clearly, before making any decisions, managers need to find out as much information as they can. The people mentioned in the case study – patients, staff, administrators, senior managers and pressure groups – are typical of those groups who may seek to influence decision-making. The decision-maker would have to consider these multiple viewpoints before allocating resources. This is obviously not easy, because these different groups all have competing interests and a vested interest in the services or programmes provided. In evaluative research such groups are often referred to as stakeholders and stakeholders may also include those providing the funding for research projects.

So what would be the role of the evaluative researcher in this process? The evaluative researcher is invaluable to the decision-making process because the researcher can provide objective information about the value of the different services provided. Although different stakeholders will all claim that their service is of value, of a researcher can assess whether this is really the case. The evaluative researcher may find that some services are ineffective or not used sufficiently by patients and may therefore suggest that such services are decreased. For example, a dietary advice clinic or a smoking cessation group which are poorly attended may be considered wasteful of valuable resources which could be re-directed elsewhere. A researcher might show that although these resources are worthwhile they may need to be delivered in a different way.

Unlike information provided by staff, patients and administrators, the findings of the researcher are relatively free from bias, because the researcher should not have a vested interest in the service provided – although we must remember that researchers working in health and social care may also have strong opinions about their work.

As distinct from other types of research, the evaluative researcher needs to work closely with stakeholders. There would be little point in the researcher deciding on a research problem in which he or she was interested unless it was relevant to the stakeholders in the area concerned. The evaluative researcher therefore needs to negotiate research questions and methods with those whose interests will be served by the researcher's work. The researcher will therefore need to ensure that questions are not formulated in such a way as to serve the interests of decision-makers rather than of client groups. The outcome of evaluative research will usually produce results which are practical rather than theoretical and which can therefore be used to influence policy decision-making.

Summary

1 In this session we have defined and discussed the process of evaluative research and applied it to health care. We also differentiated between evaluative research and exploratory research through a consideration of case material.

2 We considered the nature and design of the 'research question' in evaluative research and realised the importance of clarity in this process.

3 We explored the meanings of evaluative research within critical research methodology and recognised their importance in the wider evaluation of the caring services. Case study examples were provided as a means of illuminating this style of research methodology.

4 The session concluded by suggesting that evaluative research inclusive of critical methodology can be an important influence on policy decision-making at local and national level.

Before you move on to Session Two, check that you have achieved the objectives given at the beginning of this session and, if not, review the appropriate sections.

Qualitative and quantitative approaches to evaluative research

Introduction

This session will build on your knowledge gained from previous units about qualitative and quantitative approaches to research. As you will probably remember, all research is divided into these two categories. Evaluative research is no exception to this rule. In discussing qualitative and quantitative approaches we will move the discussion on to encompass **inductive** and **deductive** approaches to research. We will also discuss the views of different authors concerning the combining of qualitative and quantitative approaches. You will then be in a position to select an appropriate method to evaluate the services you provide.

Inductive research: *Identification of certain patterns which may lead to the formulation of hypotheses or general theories that may be tested deductively.*

Deductive research: *Research which is designed to test the validity of general theories.*

Session objectives

When you have completed this session you should be able to:

- recall the meaning of the terms qualitative and quantitative research and give examples of the methods of data collection used for each

- describe the 'black box' approach to evaluative research

- explain inductive and deductive approaches to theory development in evaluative research

- define the meaning of triangulation and explain its uses in evaluative research.

1: Which approach to use?

One of the important decisions you will need to make before carrying out evaluative research is whether to use a qualitative or quantitative approach. To review your understanding of these terms before we apply them to evaluative research and critical research methodology you should now do the following activity.

ACTIVITY 4   ALLOW 10 MINUTES

Without referring back to the other units of study in this course, write down in the spaces provided:

1 Your own definition of qualitative research and quantitative research.

2 The different methods of collecting data that would be used for each approach.

1 *Qualitative research*

Definition:

Quantitative research

Definition:

2 *Methods of collecting data for qualitative research*

Methods of collecting data for quantitative research

Commentary

1 You will probably recall that while qualitative research is concerned with assessing characteristics of people that can only be expressed through open questioning or observation, quantitative research is concerned with characteristics of people that can be assigned numerical scores which can then be counted. Asking people's opinions of a new product using open-ended questions would be an example of qualitative research, whereas asking people's height, weight and shoe size are examples of quantitative research. Observing people in their natural setting would also be an example of qualitative research.

   Allowing respondents to express their feelings in full is a qualitative measurement because a wider and deeper range of responses is likely and the researcher will use different methods (other than counting) to make sense of the findings. However, if you started to count the number of times people exhibited specific behaviours you would be quantifying the data, because this behaviour could be measured using a scale. For example, respondents could be asked to tick the box that most accurately reflected their feelings – 'sad', 'despondent', 'depressed' and 'melancholic' could be possible responses and a numerical score could be given to each one. What makes a characteristic like 'feelings' qualitative or quantitative is not always the nature of the characteristic, but the way in which it is measured.

2 You may also recall that these two approaches to study adopt different methods for collecting data, although there are overlaps between them. Qualitative methods tend to rely on:

   - interviews

   - open-ended questionnaires

   - observations

   - videos

   - tape transcripts.

   Quantitative methods, on the other hand, tend to use:

   - closed-ended questionnaires

   - rating scales

   - scientific experiments in which characteristics can be measured using a numerical score.

Before we move on to apply these two approaches to evaluative research, the next activity will further test your understanding of the nature of qualitative and quantitative approaches.

ACTIVITY 5 ALLOW 15 MINUTES

By each example below, indicate whether it is qualitative or quantitative and give your reasons why.

                                          Qualitative   Quantitative

1 A **Likert scale** with responses ranging from 'strongly agree' to 'strongly disagree' used to measure nurses' attitudes to mental illness in patients.

Likert scale: *An attitude scale which comprises a list of positively and negatively worded statements with which respondents are asked to indicate their strength of agreement or disagreement.*

19

Qualitative   Quantitative

2   Blood tests taken to measure cholesterol
    levels following the administration of
    a new drug.

3   A focus group interview used to
    ascertain the views of women about
    ante-natal care provision.

4   Children videoed in a child assessment
    centre to assess the number and type
    of disruptive behaviours.

5   The types and amount of injuries to
    children who attend an accident and
    emergency department ascertained
    by reviewing hospital records.

6   A questionnaire comprising open
    questions used to assess levels
    of coping following bereavement.

7   Participant observation used to assess
    the nature of interactions between
    health care staff and patients.
    The researcher uses field notes
    (a record of everything that happens
    and is said) to record the data.

Commentary

Answers to the above activity are as follows.

1   A Likert scale is quantitative because scores are allocated to responses from 'strongly agree' to 'strongly disagree' which are then counted. One could, however, argue that it is qualitative because it does not measure a truly quantifiable thing in the same way that a thermometer measures temperature.

2   Blood test measurements are quantitative because they provide a numerical value which will normally be subjected to statistical testing.

3   The focus group interview is qualitative because the range of responses is likely to be wide and the researcher has little control over responses.

4   Although the use of videos is often associated with qualitative research (for example when used to record naturally occurring events), their use for this purpose is quantitative because the recorded behaviours are counted and categorised. The researcher may use a scoring sheet to document each time a particular type of behaviour occurs.

5   This is quantitative because types and amount of injuries are counted.

6   The use of open questions mean that this is qualitative research. As in the focus group interview, the researcher has little control over what is said.

7   The use of field notes makes this qualitative research. Had the researcher used a coding device or scoring sheet to count the number of different types of interactions (for example, touch, gesture, verbal) this would have been quantitative research.

The examples in the activity above demonstrate two important factors in distinguishing between qualitative and quantitative approaches.

1 Quantitative researchers often use measuring tools or devices such as coding sheets to collect data. Qualitative researchers arrive at the scene armed with very little except good listening and observation skills.

2 Quantitative researchers have considerable control over responses due to the devices used – even when responses occur spontaneously researchers have control over how to code them. Qualitative researchers have very little control over events – they record what happens as it occurs and in its pure form.

This second concept, of control over data during the collection phase, is one of the main distinguishing features between qualitative and quantitative approaches. The degree of researcher control in the application of evaluative research has changed during the past few decades, with researchers moving away from controlling data collection, through experimental studies, towards more qualitative methods in which they are more receptive to naturally occurring data over which they have little control.

We have established that control over the data collection process is one difference between qualitative and quantitative methods. A third way we can distinguish between these two methods in relation to evaluative research is to look at what Chen and Rossi (1983) refer to as the 'black box'.

The black box approach to evaluation

Chen and Rossi (1983) argue that early evaluation studies which used quantitative methods were only concerned with 'input/output' evaluation. What seemed to happen was that a programme was set up which could be described as 'input' because participants were given a service which they had previously not been given. The use of parent-held records in health visiting is an example of a recent service to which parents previously did not have access. The users' responses would be measured on the relevant characteristic (such as satisfaction with existing service provision) *before* the input and then they would be measured on the same dimension *after* they had received the service. This is what Chen and Rossi describe as the 'output'. They argue that what this approach does is to create a black box in which the important elements of the programme are measured but are not analysed for their meaning.

Although this kind of research is successful in assessing whether or not the programme works, it gives no insight into transformational processes between inputs and outputs of the programme or, put simply, what has happened *inside* the black box. For example, a satisfaction score may suggest that parents are more satisfied with health visiting services since the introduction of parent-held records. However, this gives no indication of how parents and health professionals have used the records or whether they have empowered parents in any way. Swanson and Chapman (1994) point out that the results achieved through such methods often show little or no effect from an intervention even though there may have been effects.

These problems are quite worrying in health and social care because if no specific benefits are perceived by decision-makers they may withdraw the service. For example, parent held records could be withdrawn if satisfaction with the health visiting service is not seen to be specifically affected by them. Obviously, if such results are limited to purely quantitative input/output measurements, then services could be withdrawn without sufficient consideration.

The obvious solution to this problem is to use qualitative methods which seek to understand and explain what has happened in the black box (Judd, 1987). This involves an examination not only of what has happened, but how and why. Such detail is naturally more comprehensive and is a much sounder basis on which to make decisions about service provision than a simple input/output approach. This explains why contemporary evaluative research has often favoured qualitative and critical research methods rather than quantitative methods.

2: Critical research methods in evaluative research

In Session One we noted that evaluative research is more overtly political than other approaches to research because the researcher is attempting to influence policies and decisions in health and social service departments. As we have seen, it is for this reason that some approaches to evaluative research can be described as critical research methodology.

You will probably recall that in Session One we introduced four key words which underpin critical research methods. These are:

- advocacy

- activism

- empowerment

- emancipation.

These concepts are important because they represent areas of potential conflict for evaluative researchers undertaking critical research. For example, the researcher may feel a sense of loyalty towards the stakeholder who has funded the research but may also be aware that clients' needs are not being met, or that staff morale is low. The researcher then has to decide which role to adopt. For example, should he or she act as an advocate for the staff or service users or make staff or clients aware of protocols through which they could make their voices heard? The researcher must, therefore, decide at the design stage to what extent a critical research methodology approach is appropriate.

You will recall from Session One that the methodology used in critical research is qualitative because this approach offers the researcher the chance to develop a dialogue with respondents during the data collection stage. Interviews, conversations and other methods which enable the researcher to understand the world of the participants are therefore the usual method of collecting data for the critical research methodologist. However, interviews conducted in critical research are not as straightforward as one might imagine. Unlike most research in which interviews are used, critical research interviews require that the researcher get much more involved in the world of the participants in order for inequalities to be uncovered.

The interview relationship in critical research relies on three important concepts:

- a dialectical relationship

- interrogation

- exposure of the researcher's incorrect assumptions (misapprehensions).

A *dialectical* relationship refers here to the close, *two-way* interaction that needs to develop between the researcher and the subject. When we talk about *interrogation* it is the researcher's understanding that is interrogated, not the views of the respondent. This is achieved by the researcher checking with respondents that his or her interpretation is correct. By engaging in this process, any existing misapprehensions or misunderstandings on the part of the researcher are brought out into the open and explained. For example, as a researcher you may have certain misapprehensions which have developed through your own life experience. Female researchers may have different assumptions about domestic violence than those of male researchers. The researchers' assumptions may also be influenced by race or gender. Interrogation is important in ensuring that our life experiences do not unduly influence our understanding of the information presented by the respondent.

These three concepts are interrelated. An evaluative researcher conducting critical research using qualitative methods could use these approaches to gain a deeper understanding of the experience of the programme participants. This is useful because the best way to evaluate a programme is probably to experience it. Considering the experience of the users is probably as close as the researcher can realistically get to understanding this reality. A critical evaluator would probably argue that it is this reality that should be used to influence decision-makers.

We will now take a few minutes to review the main concepts discussed so far in this session and how they relate to evaluative research.

Figure 1 shows the links and contrasts between evaluative research and critical research methodology. As we have seen these two approaches to research are distinctly different from each other but share a common theme – influencing the decision-making process. Because critical research methodology is designed to seek the deeper meanings of experience with a view to transforming the future through service provision, then evaluative research could be described as a form of critical research methodology. However, as *Figure 1* also indicates, evaluative research can use a variety of approaches to data collection other than the purely qualitative approaches used in critical research. This variety, combined with the greater range of stakeholders considered in evaluative research, represents the point of departure from critical research methodology.

The evaluative researcher who chooses to use critical research methodology can use the experience of service users to demonstrate the effectiveness of service provision. It is this information that will influence decision-makers to improve services.

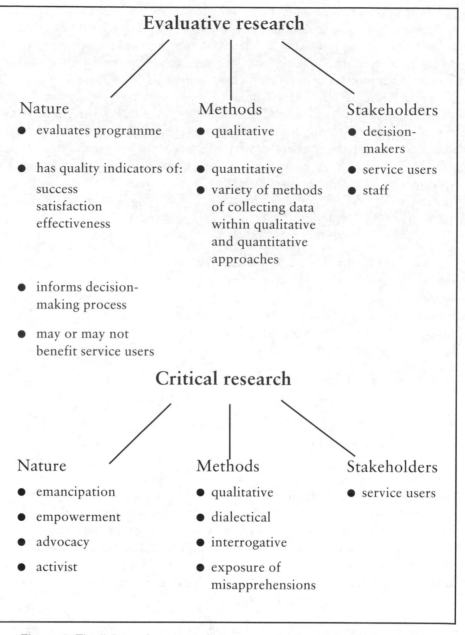

Figure 1: The links and contrasts between evaluative and critical research

At this point we need to recap our understanding of inductive and deductive approaches to evaluation.

3: Inductive and deductive approaches to evaluative research

In Unit 2 of this series, Clifford (1997) described the way theory is developed using inductive and deductive reasoning. You may recall that she described inductive reasoning as the first step in knowledge: the task of inductive reasoning is to bring knowledge into view for the first time. You may also recall from Unit 2 that deductive reasoning uses existing facts and knowledge to generate new theories. For example, a researcher may be aware of existing knowledge that suggests that people with certain chromosomal abnormalities exhibit certain characteristics. Existing knowledge may also suggest that these characteristics can be controlled using certain techniques. From this information the researcher can predict or deduce (hypothesise) that techniques applied to people with certain conditions are likely to improve the condition.

ACTIVITY 6

Read the examples of research in the case studies below and then answer the following questions.

1 Which of the two examples is inductive? Explain your answer.

2 Which of the two examples is deductive? Explain your answer.

3 Which of the two examples is qualitative? Explain your answer.

4 Which of the two examples is quantitative? Explain your answer.

Case Study 1

Orr was interested in how women have achieved change through the women's health movement and the development of women's health groups. Orr studied one such group for over three years. Rather than being based on existing knowledge, Orr's study was based on beliefs about feminism and how people perceive their situation.

Through her interaction with the group she wished to make women's experiences visible and influential in effecting changes in health care provision. Orr used a participant observation research method because she was concerned with the interrelation of subjective and objective material. She took notes during the meetings and wrote them up in more detail afterwards.

Orr's discussion of information gleaned from these meetings includes a description of the number of women who attended, the topics discussed and some of the stories told by the women.
(Orr, 1992)

Case Study 2

Dingwall and **Fox** were interested in the perennial question of whether health visitors should be nurses. This gave rise to the question of the extent to which a nursing background influences health visiting practice. Because there are several areas of overlap between the work of health visitors and social workers in relation to child mistreatment, the authors decided to examine the degree of difference in perceptions of child care problems between health visitors and social workers. The authors believed that any differences between the two occupations could be explained in terms of their different background and training.

To conduct the study the authors drew on existing knowledge by adapting a technique developed to study professional and lay definitions of child mistreatment in the United States. This technique comprised 78 pairs of vignettes depicting incidents of varying severity of child mistreatment which had been derived from professional literature and recorded cases of law and local practice. Respondents were required to define and rate each vignette as mistreatment or non-mistreatment.

The 78 pairs of vignettes were reduced to 20 by Dingwall and Fox and distributed to 20 health visitors and 20 social workers in England. The results were analysed using the mean and standard deviations as well as a t-test statistic (an inferential statistic). Interestingly, they found a lack of difference between social workers' and health visitors' perceptions of child care problems, despite the difference in background between the two groups. (Dingwall and Fox, 1992)

Commentary

1 Orr's study is inductive because she relies solely on data that emerges from her observations and her own interpretation rather than using existing facts and theories to deduce relationships. Orr does not attempt to deduce any relationships between variables based on previous research. She is only interested in the experience of the women within the context of the women's health group.

2 The second case study is deductive because Dingwall and Fox deduce relationships between variables (previous background and perceptions of child mistreatment) and use a previously developed technique to collect their data. They are using a deductive approach by relying on existing knowledge to guide their research.

3 Orr's research is qualitative because she uses participant observation to enable her to look at the interrelationship of subjective and objective information. She also uses grounded theory in the collection and analysis of data. Grounded theory involves the researcher in developing theories from data during the research process rather than beginning the research with clearly defined theoretical assumptions. This is typical of qualitative enquiry.

4 Dingwall and Fox's research is typical of quantitative research. The responses to the vignettes were calculated using both descriptive statistics (means and standard deviations) and inferential statistics (t-tests).

Now that we have reviewed the difference between inductive and deductive methods of evaluation we will go on to apply these concepts to the issue of big Q and small q questions in evaluative research.

Big Q and small q questions

One of the main distinctions between deductive and inductive approaches in evaluative research concerns the use of small q and big Q questions. According to Chen and Rossi (1983), small q questions look for answers, whereas big Q questions look for questions.

Inductive research, due to its interest in generating rather than answering questions, is asking big Q questions. The researcher is more concerned with what is going on inside the black box than with the input/output of the black box. This interest in the process rather than the outcome of the black box is typical of qualitative research. The researcher is receptive to any findings that may emerge from open questions and observations. For example, a researcher using in-depth interviews to seek understanding of people's experience of homelessness will be asking big Q questions.

Deductive research, on the other hand, is tightly controlled by the researcher and therefore asks small q questions. The researcher is only interested in what he or she can put into the black box and what will come out at the end. The richness and detail of any transformations going on inside the black box are of no interest to the deductive researcher. This is typical of the quantitative approach. The researcher studying homelessness would be more concerned with the effects of a new housing policy on the *number* of homeless people than with the way they experience their situations.

ACTIVITY 7   ALLOW 15 MINUTES

Fill in the correct terms in the table below under the correct headings.

Type of research	Type of questions	Black box	Research approach
Inductive			
Deductive			

Commentary

Your completed table should look like the one below.

Type of research	Type of questions	Black box	Research approach
Inductive	big Q questions	transformation	qualitative
Deductive	small q questions	input/output	quantitative

What relevance do these approaches to research have in health and social care settings? The next activity will help you to relate these approaches to practice.

ACTIVITY 8   ALLOW 20 MINUTES

Read the following case study and answer the questions that follow, providing reasons for your answer.

> **Sylvia** is a staff nurse on an oncology (cancer) ward. She hypothesises that pain levels of patients with terminal cancer will reduce following the use of complementary therapy. At the beginning of the research she administers a questionnaire to 20 patients suffering from terminal cancer, to assess pain levels. The questionnaire asks respondents to indicate how intense their pain is on a scale from 'severe' to 'mild'. Respondents are also asked to describe the pain in two sentences, and to state how long they have suffered the pain. After a complementary therapy technique has been delivered to the patients, Sylvia administers the same questionnaire. While the patients are undergoing the complementary therapy she monitors the patients' blood pressure and observes them for any signs of pain, such as body movements or skin pallor, which are recorded throughout. This information will show the speed with which the therapy works as well as any fluctuations in pain or side-effects of treatment during the treatment process.

1 Do you think this kind of research is evaluative research?

2 Does the research use critical research methodology?

3 Is the research deductive or inductive?

4 Are small q or big Q questions being asked?

5   Is the approach to the black box input/output or transformational?

6   Is the research qualitative or quantitative?

Commentary

1   The case study could be described as evaluative research because Sylvia is evaluating the effectiveness of something – complementary therapy.

2   The research does not use critical research methodology because Sylvia and the subjects are not engaged in a dialectical relationship and no interrogation is taking place.

3   A deductive approach is used for this research because it draws on knowledge concerning complementary therapy and people's experience of pain. On the basis of existing facts and theories Sylvia formulates an hypothesis which can then be tested.

4   The issue of big Q and small q questions is an interesting one because we could argue that in this case Sylvia is interested in both. By measuring pain at the beginning and end of the research, small q questions are asked. However the monitoring and observation of the patient during the research could lead her to ask big Q questions concerning fluctuations in pain during the therapy or the side-effects of treatment.

5   Because Sylvia is interested in both big and small q questions she is interested in both input/output issues and the transformation that takes place within the black box. The initial questionnaire represents the input, the final questionnaire represents the output, and the monitoring and recording of blood pressure and signs of pain during the research illustrates her interest in how exactly complementary therapy reduces pain.

6   The answer to the final question would depend on the type of questions Sylvia asked in the questionnaires. The questionnaires could be either quantitative or qualitative depending on whether open or closed questions were used. Clearly the monitoring of blood pressure is a quantitative measurement. The observations made during the research could be qualitative or quantitative depending on whether a coding sheet of pain categories and behaviours was used.

We can see from this activity that research which appears fairly straightforward may not in practice be quite so clear cut. In fact, research often becomes confusing in practice because we often attempt to make our research fit text-book-defined methods.

The importance of using research tools to *assist* you in research should not be understated. The trick is not to become a slave to research methods, but rather to use them for your own purposes. For example, you may read about a particular research method that you find interesting and feel tempted to look for a research problem that enables you to use this particular method. However, what you *should* do is to identify real research problems in your sphere of work and then find out which is the best research method to help you to address the problem.

You will probably find that your search for a genuine research problem still results in you defining a problem that suits your preferred approach to research. If your sympathy is with qualitative research you will probably be drawn to the type of research problems than need to be addressed using this approach. The same applies to quantitative research. You may, of course, have sympathy with both approaches and define your research question in such a way that both approaches are appropriate.

In order to help you understand the way in which research is carried out in practice, we will ask the same questions as before about a different case study.

ACTIVITY 9	ALLOW 15 MINUTES

Read the case study below and answer the questions that follow.

Mark is an AIDS specialist nurse. He is interested in the experience of people with AIDS-related illnesses and the way they perceive the support they receive from the caring professions. He is particularly interested in uncovering any problems encountered by these people and is concerned to ensure that their needs are met by the services provided. Developing a close dialectical relationship with participants is important to Mark, so that participants can be empowered to make their needs known to those with the power to allocate resources.

Mark uses participant observation as a research method by spending three hours daily for one year in a unit specialising in AIDS, during which time he observes the interaction between staff and patients. The same group of patients are interviewed in depth about their experiences of professional carers. The interviews are used to illuminate the findings from the observation and he uses the dialectical relationship to ensure that his interpretation is an accurate representation of the patients' sense of care received, rather than being based on previously held beliefs and assumptions.

---

1   Is the research evaluative research?

2 Does the research use critical research methodology?

3 Is the research deductive or inductive?

4 Are small q or big Q questions being asked?

5 Is the approach to the black box input/output or transformational?

6 Is the research qualitative or quantitative?

Commentary

The situation in this case study is more clear cut than the previous one.

1 The research is exploratory rather than evaluative. Mark, rather than evaluating a service, is exploring the field and could develop a service as a result of his findings – a service which could then be evaluated either during or following its implementation.

2 This research could be described as critical research methodology because Mark's misapprehensions concerning living with AIDS would be uncovered through interrogation. He may also take on various roles within

the relationship such as advocate or political activist or may empower the participants by providing information about resources available from certain statutory and voluntary organisations. We can see that Mark is not only collecting data. He could also help the client to improve his or her circumstances. Far from being concerned about introducing bias into the research by contaminating the data – a possible concern in the last case study – Mark could combine the role of a researcher with that of a caring professional.

3 This research is inductive rather than deductive because Mark is not drawing on existing knowledge to make generalisations about a different research area. Also, since he is carrying out in-depth interviews he is open to the suggestions and concerns of the respondents. More precise research questions will be developed as the research progresses. For example, the data may reveal that people with AIDS develop closer relationships with some professional carers than with others. Mark may then speculate about why this is so. As the research progresses it may become apparent that some professional carers have attended professional courses about AIDS. Mark may then hypothesise that:

'People suffering from AIDS-related illnesses develop closer relationships with, and are more satisfied with the care given by, staff who have attended professional courses related to AIDS than staff who have not attended such courses.'

4 & 5 It is clear that big Q questions are important to Mark. He is not interested in inputs and outputs, but in the whole experience as lived by the respondent – a big question indeed! This means that the interest in the black box is most definitely transformational.

6 The fact that Mark is using in-depth interviews makes the research qualitative.

The two case studies we have considered show very different approaches to research and demonstrate that research is not always as straightforward as it first appears. Although it is clear that some studies require a quantitative approach and others require a qualitative approach, it is often sensible to use both qualitative and quantitative methods in the same study. However, combining both of these approaches is quite a controversial issue in the research world. We will now consider the merits of combining qualitative and quantitative methods in evaluative research. We will begin with two opposing viewpoints: one which states that qualitative and quantitative methods should not be combined, and the other which states that this is entirely appropriate.

4: To combine or not to combine?

Leininger (1994) believes that mixing qualitative and quantitative methods violates the intent, purposes and philosophies of each approach. For Leininger, the distinct philosophies and purposes of these two different approaches are of central importance. Although both seek to discover the 'truth' they achieve this from different philosophical perspectives.

The purpose of the qualitative approach is to seek truth through understanding meaning in terms of the way it is understood by participants. The researcher's role here is to *interpret* the data. It is difficult for the qualitative researcher to become detached from the data and their meaning. The purpose of quantitative research is to establish truth by scientific measurements or surveys which can be recorded numerically. The quantitative researcher's role is less open to bias because no personal interpretation is expected – indeed the analysis of the data is normally undertaken by a computer which allows no room for human bias.

It is easy to see why Leininger feels the two methods should not be combined – the two philosophies are so different that it is actually counter-productive; but how do we resolve the problem that in reality we may need to collect both quantitative and qualitative information in order to gain a more complete understanding of the situation? In fact, a more complete understanding arrived at by combining both methods may be the closest we can get to actually establishing the 'truth'. We will now consider the alternative viewpoint.

Evaluative research is concerned with seeking the views of different stakeholders in order to evaluate service provision accurately. This need to take multiple perspectives into account can be addressed by combining both quantitative and qualitative methods within the evaluation design. Mullen and Iverson (1986) suggest that quantitative methods *confirm* or *verify* theory, whereas qualitative methods *discover* theory. This means that while the researcher may begin with a theory about the effectiveness of a programme which can be confirmed or verified quantitatively, qualitative methods then need to be used to discover new theories about what is happening to the users of the service. Swanson and Chapman (1994) describe this as 'exploring the multiple realities of the actors in a changing social scene by engaging them in dialogue and being open to their interpretations of the world'.

Reichardt and Cook (1979) believe that for evaluation to be comprehensive it must be both process- and outcome-oriented, exploratory and confirmatory – in other words, that qualitative and quantitative methods should be combined. Guba and Lincoln (1989) and Patton (1986, 1987) also recommend combining qualitative and quantitative methods in evaluative research.

As you can see, there are convincing arguments for combining both approaches to evaluation. We will now explore the term 'triangulation' which explains how a combination of both approaches is actually carried out.

Triangulation

Triangulation refers to the combining of different methodologies in the study of the same phenomenon (Denzin, 1978). Denzin referred to two approaches to triangulation:

- between-methods triangulation

- within-method triangulation.

'Between-methods triangulation' refers to combining methods of data collection *between* the two approaches to research. Examples of this would be combining in-depth interviews (qualitative) with a survey questionnaire comprised of closed questions (quantitative). The advantage of combining both methods would be to test the degree of 'external validity' – that is, how much the results can be generalised to other populations. If the results converge (agree with each other) we can be more certain that they are an accurate depiction of the truth. The following case study illustrates this approach.

Between-methods triangulation

As publishers we are interested in how satisfied you are with your learning as a result of studying this package. We decide to use a triangulation approach by distributing closed-ended questionnaires (quantitative) to a sample of students who have used these materials and selecting a sample of the respondents for an in-depth interview (qualitative). The fact that we are combining a quantitative questionnaire with a qualitative interview makes this research an example of between-methods triangulation.

Convergence: This occurs when two methods of research produce the same results.

Respondents may tell us different things during the interview from those they put on the questionnaire, or the findings from the interview and the questionnaire may support each other. If there is a good degree of **convergence** then we will feel quite satisfied that the findings are pretty typical of all students studying these materials. If most students make the same suggestions for improvement we can feel confident in making the necessary changes. However, if students tell us different things in the interview to what they said in the questionnaire we become less sure of our findings and will need to collect more data until we become more certain.

'Within-method triangulation' refers to the use of different methods of collecting data *within* one general approach. For example, within the qualitative approach participant observation could be used to understand the interactions between a group of people. This could then be supported by interviews to find out whether the researcher's interpretations were accurate. The following case study illustrates how this approach may be used.

Within-method triangulation

Irene is an occupational therapist who specialises in mental health problems. Part of her job involves running group therapy sessions for patients. She has decided to conduct an exploratory study to gain a better understanding of the type of interactions that happen in the group. This understanding will enable her to understand the needs of her patients better so that she can plan her sessions more effectively.

She decides to use a triangulation approach by combining observation with in-depth interviews. The qualitative nature of the approach requires that all interactions are recorded as they occur (observations) rather than using a coding system. Triangulation occurs when Irene checks the accuracy of her understanding of the data using in-depth interviews (another form of qualitative approach) to ask people whether what she thought was happening in the group agreed with what they thought was happening. This helps to ensure that her initial understanding of her observations is accurate and therefore reliable. Because Irene is combining two qualitative methods, this is known as 'within-method triangulation'.

Jick (1979) argues that triangulation can uncover unique characteristics of the participants which the participants themselves are insufficiently aware of to reveal and which might have been neglected had a single method been used. Jick refers to this as 'illumination of context' because deeper dimensions of the participants emerge and the researcher's understanding is enriched.

Another advantage of triangulation, according to Jick, is that it builds on the strengths of the different methods and therefore neutralises the problems that may occur when a single method is used. For example, sending questionnaires to students studying this package might only reveal very superficial information which could create a false impression of their experience. Interviewing a small sample of these students could add a depth of information lacking in the questionnaires. Survey research using questionnaires could, therefore, give us more confidence in the results of a small sample of qualitative in-depth interviews and qualitative methods could help to shed light on findings from quantitative research.

Summary

1   In this session we have discussed the value of both qualitative and quantitative approaches to evaluative research and considered opposing arguments about combining these two approaches.

2   We have discussed inductive and deductive approaches to theory development and have considered these in the light of big Q and small q questions.

3   We have defined the meaning of triangulation and explained its uses in evaluative research.

Before you move on to Session Three, check that you have achieved the objectives given at the beginning of this session and, if not, review the appropriate sections.

SESSION THREE

Design issues in evaluative research

Introduction

In addition to selecting qualitative or quantitative approaches for their research, researchers need to make another important decision. They need to choose between formative and summative evaluation designs and define their methodology further by selecting either an experimental or non-experimental design. This session will guide you through this process.

Before we begin this session it is worth distinguishing between the terms 'research *approach*' and 'research *design*'. Research approach refers to the overall philosophical approach that underpins the way the research is carried out, for example, qualitative and quantitative approaches. Research design refers to the way the research is planned, including control of variables, designing instruments for collecting data and managing the data-collection process.

Session objectives

When you have completed this session you should be able to:

- distinguish between formative and summative designs in evaluative research

- distinguish between experimental and quasi-experimental designs in evaluative research

- understand the notations used in experimental and quasi-experimental designs

- explain how to design a research study to establish the value of a programme.

1: Formative and summative approaches to evaluation

We need to start by establishing what is meant by the terms 'summative' and 'formative'. You may have come across these terms in the educational field when they are used in relation to assignments. Students can be required to produce formative assignments and summative assignments, for example.

Formative refers to measurements or assessments which are not actually used as part of an overall final score or grade, but which give an indication of progress at some point during the programme. Formative essays, also referred to as diagnostic essays, are designed to give students feedback about their performance without the threat and anxiety of the scores being used to determine their final pass grade. Formative can therefore be said to be ongoing assessment used *throughout* rather than at the *end* of a programme, the results of which have no bearing on the final score.

Summative, on the other hand, refers to measurements which take place at the end of a programme. You may have been subjected to summative assignments at the end of a programme of study. These results are always important because they are the final outcome of your study and determine a pass or fail.

Applying these concepts to evaluative research, formative evaluation refers to continuous feedback *during the course* of the programme evaluation which involves stage-by-stage comparison between stated objectives and what is actually being achieved (Phillips et al., 1994). The emphasis is therefore on evaluation in order to *improve* the programme (Popham, 1993). As Thorpe (1988) points out, formative evaluation asks questions like 'how are we doing?' and 'what should we be doing next?' Thorpe believes that the emphasis is on identifying changes which need to be made to improve the programme and help it achieve its goals, rather than on measuring effectiveness. Formative evaluation is concerned with how well goals are being achieved, rather than with whether they were the right goals in the first place.

Phillips et al. (1994) define summative evaluation as evaluation which takes place after the programme has finished. The emphasis here is on whether or not to continue (Popham, 1993) and with assessing the effectiveness of the completed programme. Summative evaluation asks questions like 'were the aims achieved?', 'was it worth doing?' and 'is it worth continuing?' (Thorpe, 1988).

Thorpe (1988) describes a spectrum of evaluative research with summative evaluation at one end and formative evaluation at the other. The main characteristics of formative and summative evaluations are as follows.

Formative evaluation:

- occurs during the programme and responds to concerns as they arise within the programme

- is performed by the health practitioner, often as part of his or her work

- is relatively inexpensive due to its reliance on existing staff

- is small scale and may use descriptive statistics or qualitative analysis

- tends to be reported within local health authority trusts or social services departments

- is driven by the concerns of decision-makers and the operational constraints of the organisation: decision-makers may, in the interests of organisational efficiency, demand a research method which may not portray an accurate account of the subject of the study

- is interested in *monitoring* performance indicators or short-term effects of the programme on patient/client care and allows the researcher to continually feed the research findings into the decision-making process.

Summative evaluation:

- occurs at the end of the programme in that a final research report is produced

- uses specialist outside evaluators because the evaluation is often large-scale and needs to be accurate

- is costly in time and resources because of the expertise required

- tends to use large-scale surveys or experiments requiring inferential statistical analysis due to the need for accuracy

- may be funded by, and reported nationally through, major reports published by professional organisations such as the National Association of Health Authorities and Trusts

- is driven by methodological concerns such as the need for a representative sample and a strong research design

- is interested in the long-term effects of the programme on patient/client care.

Thorpe (1988) argues that because results are important in a summative evaluation and could determine the future of the programme, a truly representative sample of the population is essential and data collection needs to be comprehensive. In formative evaluation, however, since findings are temporary and merely provide indications of progress, instant feedback can be given to practitioners and service providers so that ongoing changes to the programme can be made. Polit and Hungler (1987) refer to formative evaluation as using 'loose' methods because suggestions for improvement can come from:

- unstructured discussions with relevant individuals

- informal observations of the programme in operation

- an individual 'armchair analysis' of materials and objectives.

For example, a researcher interested in the effectiveness of care in the community of people with mental health problems could:

- discuss the nature of the services provided with groups of staff

- interview clients about their satisfaction with the services provided

- observe group therapy sessions in day-care centres

- analyse the programme objectives in order to establish whether they have been achieved

- read records indicating types and frequency of treatment interventions.

All this might seem to suggest that formative evaluation is easier than summative evaluation because there are fewer restrictions regarding methodology. However, this is not always the case. Decision-makers are often closely involved with formative evaluators and may place restrictions on the methodology because they are funding the research and want speedy results.

We will now look at how each of these approaches could be used for the same research problem.

Formative evaluation

Sandy is a paediatric nurse who has decided to develop a new programme in which children about to be admitted to hospital for surgery attend a Saturday morning club at the hospital. The club is a chance for the children to meet nursing staff and be introduced to the ward environment and play area. Sandy decides to evaluate the effectiveness of the programme formatively so that the responses of the children and their parents can be monitored and any suggestions for improvement implemented immediately. Sandy uses the following research methods:

- observation of the children for signs of distress or signs of positive behaviour indicating that the children are enjoying the club

- questionnaires distributed to parents to assess whether they felt that the club had helped in reducing their child's anxiety about the idea of coming into hospital

- assessment of the children throughout their stay in hospital to see whether the club had been effective in helping them to adjust to hospitalisation.

Sandy involves all staff, including non-specialist , less-trained staff, in the observation and questioning and ensures that all staff understand how to observe the children and administer the questionnaire. Throughout the process Sandy informs her manager of any progress made. Her manager has given the project her approval but is concerned about the time required to collect the data. Sandy therefore needs to obtain results quickly so that her manager can make a decision regarding the future of the club. If Sandy does not collect her data quickly and with minimum disruption to the ward routine she may be forced by her manager to abandon the project.

Sandy has made a conscious decision to use a formative evaluation design, rather than a summative design, despite its weaknesses. She has probably accepted these weaknesses because the research is small-scale and she really only wants to gain an impression of the value of the club during the early stages of its development so that prompt changes can be made.

You may have realised that there is a potential flaw in the research design of this case study. We have no yardstick against which to measure the children's response to hospitalisation because:

- we can't define what is a normal level of anxiety exhibited by children before and after an operation

- we cannot be sure that it is the Saturday morning club that reduced the anxiety levels.

A way of addressing these problems is to randomly allocate children either to a group which attends the Saturday morning club or to another group that has no such intervention. The two groups of children could then be observed to see whether the Saturday morning club group (the experimental group) appeared less anxious than the control group. A validated scale could also be used to accurately measure the anxiety levels of the children.

This latter approach to evaluation is more scientific and potentially more expensive due to the need to use validated measuring scales which might require specific research expertise. For this reason the researcher needs to decide whether a less costly formative evaluation is sufficient for the research requirements.

We will now use the Saturday morning club in another case study to demonstrate how different approaches to evaluation can be used to address the same research problem.

Summative evaluation

Sandy decides to make her research design stronger by carrying out a summative evaluation. She uses the same measurements (observations and questionnaires) but needs to be more strict in ensuring that:

- the sample is large enough

- the children are randomly allocated between the two groups

- the measuring instruments, such as assessment tools, observation sheets and questionnaires, are valid and accurately measure what they are intended to measure.

The random allocation of the children to two groups makes this an example of an experimental design which is often used in summative evaluations. Sandy uses monitoring for a different purpose in this approach. In the formative evaluation, Sandy uses monitoring to feed information back to the ward manager constantly so that changes can be made to the Saturday morning club at any stage of the research. In the summative evaluation, Sandy uses monitoring methods such as random allocation to build up a more accurate and comprehensive picture of the children's behaviour so that the results will be more reliable. She is interested in the reliability of the final report rather than using findings to change the programme as it develops. Because Sandy needs her measurements to be accurate, she may require outside assistance from researchers trained in observation techniques, rather than using existing staff who are not trained in these procedures. For this reason, before she commences the project she applies for research funding from several large organisations, including the English National Board for Nursing, Midwifery and Health Visiting (ENB) and a research scholarship advertised in a nursing journal.

The two case studies about Sandy show how two different approaches can be used for the same research problem, depending on the purpose of the enquiry. The purpose of Sandy's formative research study was to monitor the progress of and make any necessary changes to the Saturday morning club during its development. Her summative evaluation however, was more concerned with the end product and with designing a strong research methodology. Her purpose here was to provide a summative report which would help to decide whether the club should be continued or not in the light of the measured effects on the children.

ACTIVITY 10   ALLOW 15 MINUTES

1 Looking through the material given so far in this session write down examples of the kind of questions which would be asked by researchers in the Saturday morning club using:

a) the formative approach

b) the summative approach.

2 Give examples of how this scenario matches the characteristics identified by Thorpe for each kind of approach.

Commentary

1. a) The formative approach is concerned with questions like 'How is the club doing?' and 'Should we be making any changes to the club in response to concerns of parents or staff?' The researcher here is concerned with how well goals are being achieved rather than with whether they were the right ones in the first place.

    b) The summative evaluator would ask questions such as 'Did the club help reduce children's anxiety about going into hospital?', 'Is the club successful?' or 'Is it worth continuing with the club?' (Thorpe, 1988).

2. The first case study about Sandy illustrated the following features of formative evaluation.

Formative evaluation:

- occurs during the programme and responds to concerns as they arise. Sandy was gathering data in quite an informal manner

- is performed by the health practitioner, often as part of his or her work. Sandy carried out her formative evaluation as part of her job

- is relatively inexpensive due to its reliance on existing staff. The only staff that Sandy used were the existing ward staff who she ensured were able to assess children adequately

- is small scale and may use descriptive statistics or qualitative analysis. Sandy would use descriptive statistics to analyse the data from the parental questionnaires and would use qualitative data analysis to interpret her observations

- tends to be reported within local health authority trusts or social services departments. Sandy's evaluation would probably only be reported within the hospital

- is driven by the concerns of decision-makers and operational constraints of the organisation.Sandy's manager wanted quick results and was unable to provide funds to carry out a large-scale study. The evaluation was therefore driven by resource constraints – which probably produced less accurate results than would be achieved through a summative evaluation

- is interested in *monitoring* performance indicators of short-term effects of programmes on patient/client care. Monitoring the effects of the club was important to Sally because she was able to report continually to her manager the beneficial effects of the club, as well as any potential problems, as they occurred.

The second case study about Sandy illustrates the following features of summative evaluation.

Summative evaluation:

- occurs at the end of the programme. Sandy was more interested in the outcomes of the programme than the actual experience of running the programme

- uses specialist outside evaluators. This is why Sandy would seek expert advice from researchers to assist her in designing the study in a manner that would ensure accurate results

- is costly in time and resources. Sandy therefore applied for research funding to support the study

- tends to use large-scale surveys or experiments requiring inferential statistical analysis. Sandy's experimental design and use of anxiety scales would produce scores which could be subjected to statistical tests

- may be funded by, and reported nationally through, major reports published by professional organisations such as the National Association of Health Authorities and Trusts. If Sandy is awarded research funding a final report would be essential and would probably be reported nationally

- is driven by methodological concerns such as the need for a representative sample and a strong research design. Sandy randomly allocated the children to two groups and used a validated instrument for data collection to ensure that the research design was strong

- is interested in the long-term effects of the programme on patient/client care. The conclusions of Sandy's study would either result in the continuation or closure of the club and would therefore have long-term effects on the preparation of children for surgery.

Now that we have discussed formative and summative evaluation in some detail we can identify the advantages of each.

Probably the most valuable characteristics of formative evaluation are:

- its cost effectiveness

- the involvement of decision-makers and practitioners, which ensures that the research is relevant to client care

- its reliance on continual monitoring of performance.

In contrast, summative evaluation benefits from:

- a stronger methodology which produces more credible findings

- the interest in the long-term effects of a programme rather than its immediate effects

- reporting of the findings as part of national projects funded by large organisations, which ensures that the research has a high profile and good credibility.

We will now apply formative and summative evaluative methods to your own field of work.

ACTIVITY 11 — ALLOW 20 MINUTES

Write in the box below an example of formative evaluation and an example of summative evaluation that would apply to your own area of practice.

Formative evaluation

Summative evaluation

Commentary

Since your example will be very specific to your area of practice we cannot comment on what you may have written. You should, therefore, share your examples with other students, a tutor or a mentor.

2: Experimental and quasi-experimental approaches to evaluative research

We will now consider two further approaches for carrying out evaluative research – 'experimental' and 'quasi-experimental' designs. These two designs can be used within both formative and summative approaches, but tend to be used in summative evaluation designs more frequently. *Figure 2* shows how these two methods can be used within the two approaches.

Experimental research: *The collection of data in highly controlled situations.*

Quasi-experimental research: *An alternative to experimental research with many of the advantages of the experimental method. Through manipulation of the independent variable control is exerted over the study. The researcher cannot randomly allocate the subjects to an experimental and control group.*

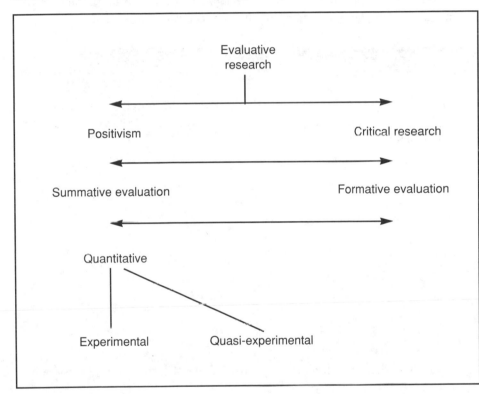

Figure 2: The continuum of research approaches used within evaluative research

The experimental approach

According to Polit and Hungler (1987) experimental research has three characteristics.

1   The researcher manipulates the independent variable.

2   There is random allocation of subjects to groups.

3   The variables that may account for the differences between the two groups are controlled to prevent bias.

A typical example of the experimental method is the 'randomised control trial', so-called because:

- subjects are *randomly* allocated between an experimental group and a control group

- any variables such as age, gender or health status that may distort the results are controlled.

Woodward (1992) suggests that the randomised control trial is considered to be the design of choice in health care when trying to assess the effectiveness of treatment. This is because, as far as possible, any variables that may account for the research findings are controlled to prevent bias. Researchers can therefore be more confident that any changes, for example, health status, are a result of the intervention rather than of other factors.

Because of the scientific nature of true experimental designs, they are often associated with medical research such as drug trials. More recently, particularly during the 1980s and 1990s, nurses have also become involved in carrying out experiments. These usually either demonstrate the effectiveness of particular types of intervention (such as dietary advice) or compare the efficacy of one treatment with another (for example, different types of dressings).

ACTIVITY 12   ALLOW 15 MINUTES

1 List two examples in which you think that a randomised control trial could be used to evaluate the effectiveness of treatment or to compare one treatment with another.

a)

b)

2 State whether you think a randomised control trial could be classified as formative or summative evaluation.

Commentary

As your own example will be specifically related to your particular sphere of practice you will need to discuss it with other students, colleagues, a tutor or a mentor. However, some additional examples follow.

1 a) Two different types of dressing (one already in use and one new one) could be applied to leg ulcers to ascertain which is the most effective in wound healing. Controls would need to be used to ensure that it was not the characteristics of the patients, such as age or health status, which were responsible for the healing rather than the type of dressing used. Half the patients would be randomly assigned to the experimental group in which the new dressing would be used. The other half would be randomly allocated to the control and would continue with the existing treatment.

b) A practice nurse might be interested in the effectiveness of a patient asthma-education programme on the control of asthma symptoms. In order to measure the effectiveness of the programme, the nurse may randomly allocate half the patients to the education programme and the other half of the patients would continue with their usual treatment. Random allocation would go some way towards ensuring that patients with asthma of differing severity, and of different ages, were equally distributed between the two groups. Peak expiratory flow measurements (the biggest 'fastest huff' a patient can produce after taking a deep breath) could be used as well as blood tests before the programme to record **baseline data** for *both* groups. The same measurements would then be recorded at the end of the programme to establish whether the patients who had received the programme had made greater improvements in controlling their asthma than those in the control group.

2 Because they are small-scale and carried out by health practitioners, the programmes in our examples of randomised control trials might appear to be formative evaluations. However, due to the need to control unwanted influences (extraneous variables) and ensure accurate research findings, the researcher is unable here to change the programme during the implementation. For example, although interviews with patients might reveal the inconvenience they experienced as a result of the intervention, the researcher is unable to respond by changing the programme because to do so might limit the effectiveness of the experiment and bias the results. (Of course, in circumstances of severe inconvenience the practitioner would be bound by professional responsibility to change the programme, but this will be a professional decision rather than a research one.)

We must conclude, then, that the inability to use the research findings to feed back into the programme at any stage makes experimental methods more typical of summative rather than formative evaluation. The writing of a research report at the end of the experiment, stating the results of the intervention and the likely benefits and costs is also typical of summative research.

Baseline data: *Data recorded before any experimental changes are made.*

Although randomised control trials are invaluable in determining the effectiveness of specific treatments, they are of limited use in other areas (such as the experience of living with AIDS) because they are concerned mainly with inputs (interventions) and outputs (effectiveness of treatment), rather than with how the patient or client *feels* about the treatment concerned. In both of the examples in the commentary above, the patients may have been subjected to inconvenience in order for the research to be carried out. The patients with the leg ulcers may have experienced some discomfort because the new dressing was of a different texture to the old dressing. In the asthma example, the patients who attended the education programme might be inconvenienced by having to be more aware of their symptoms and how to control them.

Although the use of experimental designs can result in important findings, these findings may have little impact on the long-term improvement of health status if we don't understand what patients feel about treatments.

We can think of this in terms of the black box, the contents of which are often sadly lacking in experimental designs. You may also have noticed that we are asking small q rather than big Q questions in these examples because the research is tightly controlled and interested in outcomes. One way of finding out the contents of the black box would be to use a questionnaire or interview to find out what the patients felt about the programme.

We can see that although randomised control trials are powerful research designs because of their high degree of reliability and validity, they may not be feasible to use because of ethical problems. These include depriving the control group of the intervention that the experimental group is receiving or causing discomfort for the patient. Researchers might decide whether an experimental approach is still desirable despite these limitations because the research findings will have long-term benefits that outweigh any ethical concerns.

There is another problem which experimental researchers need to plan for – that of 'contamination'. Contamination from other variables will reduce the reliability of the research to the extent that the less control there is over the experiment, the less it can be described as *true* experimental research. A researcher's ideal would be to contain the patients in a laboratory for the entire period of the study, but ethical issues would naturally preclude this! It would probably be possible for a practice nurse to measure the effectiveness of an asthma education group by randomly allocating patients to a patient education group and a control group and by making peak flow measurements. However, they would also need to measure the patients' perceptions of the group and to monitor extraneous variables that could contaminate research, for example, patients following advice from other sources such as the media or their GP.

These are two reasons why health and social care researchers often opt for an alternative to experimental research, but one which still has many of the advantages of experimental research. This alternative is called 'quasi-experimental research'.

Quasi-experimental research

Quasi-experimental research shares the first of the characteristics of experimental research (manipulation), but lacks either randomisation or control. It is therefore more difficult to make causal inferences such as 'was reduced stress in a patient the result of attending a stress group or of other factors?' Looking at the asthma education group example above, it can be seen that:

- *manipulation* of the independent variable (IV) – attendance at the group – can be achieved by allocating patients to the education group or the control group

- *randomisation* can be achieved by using a random number table so that each patient stands an equal chance of being allocated to either group

- *control* is a little more difficult to achieve due to extraneous issues (such as the effect of the media and other influences) and this is one factor that could result in this research being approached in a quasi-experimental way.

The use of a quasi-experimental approach is shown in the following case study.

Quasi-experimental research design

Sonia is a hospital manager in a large district hospital in which a new, controversial shift work pattern for staff is about to be introduced. There has already been considerable dissent among staff, but the managerial board believes that the new system will be more efficient and will save money.

Sonia is concerned about the effect that the new system will have on staff morale and therefore gains the agreement of the management board to run a six-month pilot trial in three wards before the new system is implemented.

Sonia is worried that low staff morale resulting from the new system may result in:

- an increase in sick leave
- an increase in the number of staff leaving.

She therefore looks at staff sickness records for the whole hospital for the six months prior to the introduction of the new system and continues to do so during the six months of the pilot scheme. She also examines records for staff turnover across the hospital.

Sonia then compares the wards in which the new system has been introduced with the wards that remain the same, in terms of:

- the fluctuations in sick leave during the specified period
- the number of staff leaving to take up posts elsewhere.

If absence through sickness in the staff affected by the new system goes up during the trial period, but remains the same in the other staff, and if more staff in the affected wards leave to work elsewhere, then Sonia will be able to argue that the new system is not cost effective.

Quasi-experimental research is often used for ethical reasons concerning random allocation or control of variables. In the above case study, for example, Sonia would ideally control the experiment by randomly allocating staff to the wards affected by the new system (the experimental group) and other wards (control group). This would help to control extraneous variables (unwanted influences) such as the fact that morale may differ between certain wards due to factors such as relationships between staff and the type of duties required. However, random allocation would be unethical here, partly because of the disruption to staff, but more importantly because of the impact that this might have on patient care. The disruption of staff might itself cause low staff morale, and Sonia would not know whether sickness levels were due to staff being allocated to a new ward against their will (for the experiment), or to the new shift system that the experiment was designed to assess.

In the case study, an alternative to random allocation (in which a *control* group is used) is the use of a naturally occurring *comparison* group. This means that Sonia would use all the other wards in the hospital (which are unaffected by the new system) as a comparison group with which she can compare the experimental group. However, as you may have deduced, the use of a comparison group is a less powerful design than using a control group because the subjects (staff) have not been randomly allocated between the two groups. This means that the characteristics of subjects which may affect the results (such as age, length of time qualified, family commitments, type of experience) are not equally distributed between the two groups.

For example, one ward in the experimental group might have a high proportion of female staff who are mothers of young children and who are particularly adversely affected by the new shift system. Conversely, a ward in the comparison group may have a high proportion of young, newly qualified nurses whose lifestyle is not adversely affected by the new system. The results could therefore reflect natural differences between groups rather than the changes made.

ACTIVITY 13   ALLOW 10 MINUTES

Think about the asthma education example above and try to think of an ethical problem which could cause this research design to be changed to a quasi-experimental approach.

Commentary

If some of the asthma patients are being deprived of a potential benefit (in this case, education) because they were randomly selected, an ethical problem could arise. An ethics committee could reject the proposal and insist that the researcher compare the patients with others in a different practice which does not provide an asthma education programme, so that they are not deliberately being deprived of a service by the researcher. In this case a comparison group would be used instead of a control group, thus protecting the patients' ethical rights, but reducing the power of the design.

As in Sonia's situation, subjects in comparison groups may differ on some important characteristic such as age, gender, experience etc. which could affect the results of the study. We can never be absolutely sure in a quasi-experimental design whether the changes arising from the intervention were as a result of the intervention or because of the individual characteristics of the subjects. Control then, is the essence of the difference between experimental and quasi-experimental designs.

Notation used in experimental and quasi-experimental designs

In different research textbooks you will always see the same notation used in experimental or quasi-experimental research. We will be using this in our examples.

R   =   randomisation

O   =   observation

X   =   experiment.

- *Randomisation* refers to the random allocation of subjects to the two different groups: the experimental group (also known as 'treatment or intervention group') and the control group. Random allocation is achieved most accurately using a random number table (which allocates numbers randomly to subjects) to eliminate any bias in sample selection. If the researcher merely numbered subjects from one to thirty and then placed the first fifteen in the experimental group, she or he would probably know who was being allocated to which group. The researcher might know that the first fifteen subjects are, for example, more co-operative and this itself could influence the results. True random allocation means that the researcher has no control over who gets allocated to the experimental group and the control group.

- *Observation* refers to the *measurements* taken at the different stages of the research, such as blood pressure records, blood tests, the administration of a questionnaire or the recording of certain behaviours on an observation schedule. Observations can be made at different stages of the intervention so that comparisons can be drawn between the experimental group and control group. Observations made at different time have different terms:

   pre-tests are used as a baseline measurement *before* the intervention

   mid-tests are made *half-way* through the intervention

   post-tests are made *after* the intervention

   retention tests are made a *considerable time after* the intervention to see if any benefits have been retained over time.

- *Experiment* refers to the actual experiment or intervention that is being used, such as a new drug, a new shift system or a health education programme.

The case study shown below demonstrates the way these notations are used in a typical experimental design. The **R** in the notation shows that the subjects in the case study have been randomly allocated between the experimental group and the control group.

The notation we use in the case study is:

R	experimental group	0_1		0_2
			X	
	control group	0_1		0_2

The top line shows that:

- the experimental group has an observation (pre-test 0_1) before the intervention

- the intervention is given – **X**

- a second observation is made (post-test 0_2) which can be compared with the pre-test 0_1 to see if any changes have taken place as a result of the intervention.

The bottom line shows that:

- the control group are also given a pre-test 0_1

- unlike the experimental group they are not given an intervention

- like the experimental group they are given a post-test 0_2 which can be compared with the pre-test 0_1 .

Experimental design

Sheila is a district nurse who has persuaded the GP with whom she works to prescribe a new wound dressing which, according to the manufacturers, is more effective than the usual dressings. The GP is reluctant to prescribe them because the dressing is costly, but Sheila assures her that she will conduct an experiment to compare the different dressings. Sheila uses the following notation to inform the design of her experiment:

R	experimental group	0_1		0_2
	control group	0_1	X	0_2

First, she looks through all her records for all patients on her list who need daily dressings for leg ulcers. This is her first control of the experiment. If she uses patients with different types of wounds, some of which have healed sufficiently to need dressing on alternate days, she will not know whether they have healed more quickly because of the dressing or because they were healing successfully anyway. She also restricts her sample to people of a similar age group because age is also an extraneous variable which may affect the rate of healing. Ideally, she would like all her sample to have a similar diet (this being another extraneous variable), but she realises that this would be difficult to control.

Having found a sample of thirty patients, Sheila then allocates fifteen of them to the experimental group and fifteen to the control group. She does this using a random number table (**R**).

Sheila then makes her first observation (pre-test or 0_1) of all the sample and then records the condition of the wounds, including size, colour and depth. With the permission of the patients she also photographs each wound.

She then dresses the wounds of all her patients on a daily basis. The wounds of the experimental group (**X**) patients are dressed with the 'new' dressing and the control group patients are dressed with the 'old' dressing.

After three weeks Sheila carries out a post-test (0_2). If any patients have healed during the study period Sheila documents the date that the wound healed.

Sheila then compares the rate of healing of the two groups of patients and uses a statistical software package available through her employer to calculate whether the findings were significant.

We will now apply the same notation to the following activity. The notation is:

R	experimental group	0_1		02
	control group	0_1	X	0_2

ACTIVITY 14   ALLOW 5 MINUTES

A school nurse wants to evaluate the effectiveness of a health education session given to high school pupils about AIDS and HIV. He randomly allocates the pupils to an intervention group and a control group and uses a pre-test/post test design comprising a knowledge-based test.

If the intervention was successful, i.e. the knowledge of the intervention group about AIDS increased:

1   What difference would the school nurse find between the pre-test and post-test scores in the experimental group?

2   What difference would the nurse find between the pre-test and post-test scores in the control group?

3   What difference would the nurse find between the post-test scores of each group?

Commentary

1   The nurse would find an improvement between the pre-test and post-test in the experimental group.

2   The nurse would find less improvement between the pre-test and post-test in the control group.

3   The nurse would find that the intervention group achieved higher scores than the control group at the post-test.

You now know that the two differences between experimental and quasi-experimental designs are that:

1   the experimental design uses random allocation, whereas the quasi-experiment does not

2   the experimental design uses a control group, whereas the quasi-experiment uses a comparison group.

The two similarities between the designs are:

1   both designs give the intervention (X) to the experimental group and not to the control or comparison group

2   both designs take two sets of measurements, before (0_1) and after (0_2) the intervention.

We can now return to our earlier diagram of research methodology (*Figure 2*) and insert the different designs that we have now discussed. These are represented in *Figure 3*.

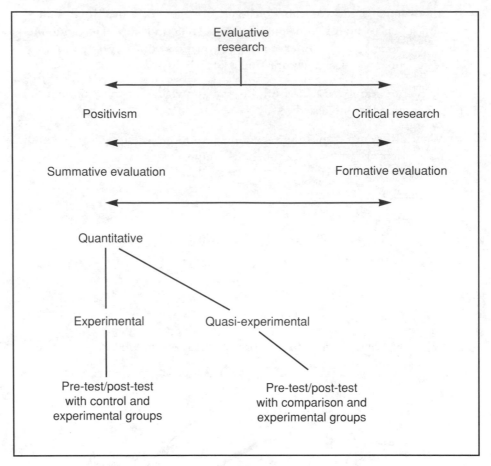

Figure 3: Different designs used for quantitative evaluation

Pre-test/post-test designs without a control group

There may be occasions when a researcher is actually unable to use either a control group or a comparison group because a similar group for comparison does not exist. For example, if new shift patterns were introduced throughout a whole hospital rather than on a small number of wards, a comparison between wards could not be made. Of course, it might be possible to compare staff morale in this hospital with staff morale in another hospital which uses a different shift pattern, but there are likely to be many factors related to the characteristics of the different hospitals, as well as shift patterns, which could affect staff morale.

In this situation it would probably be best to use a pre-test /post-test design without a control group. The lack of control group makes this a less powerful design, but some comparisons can be made between indicators of morale (such as sickness and staff turnover) before the change in shift patterns (the intervention) and after the intervention.

Because only one group is used and they are exposed to a pre-test (0_1) which acts as a baseline measurement, the intervention (X) is then given and is followed by a post-test (0_2) which can then be compared with the pre-test.

The notation used for a pre-test/post-test design is as follows:

$$0_1 \qquad X \qquad 0_2$$

The two differences between an experimental design and a pre-test/post-test design are that:

1   in the pre-test/post-test design there is no random allocation of subjects to two groups

2   in the experimental design (see notation used in case study above) a control group is used.

The similarities between the two designs are that:

1   both use two sets of observations (0_1 and 0_2)

2   both use some type of intervention (**X**).

The pre-test/post-test design is a quasi-experimental rather than an experimental design because it fulfils only two of the three criteria for an experiment. The researcher *manipulates* the independent variable, for example, the use of new shift patterns (the intervention) by imposing it on the staff. The researcher also exerts some control over the experiment. He decides what measurements to use (such as sickness rates and staff turnover), when to take measurements and whether or not to exclude certain types of staff if they are likely to bias the results (for example, those on long-term sickness which commenced before the new system was introduced). However, if the new system is introduced throughout all wards, the researcher cannot use *random allocation* and so the randomisation criteria is not met.

ACTIVITY 15   ALLOW 10 MINUTES

Read the case study below and then answer the question that follows.

A pre-test/post-test design is to be used in the measurement of satisfaction levels of patients who are receiving a district nursing service for which 'timed visits' are to be introduced. The district nurse will administer a satisfaction questionnaire to patients who have been receiving a 'non-timed' district nursing service *before* the new service (intervention) commences. The same questionnaire will then be administered *after* they have experienced the new service for a specified period of time. The district nurse will then calculate the scores for both satisfaction measurements to see if there is any difference between them. If the 'timed-visiting' service is successful the nurse would expect to find an increase in satisfaction at the post-test. This could then be used as evidence that the new system is effective and therefore worth continuing.

What do you think the limitation of this design would be?

Commentary

The measurements (satisfaction levels) fail to acknowledge that something else other than the intervention could be responsible for the change in satisfaction at the end of the programme. Characteristics such as age, gender or experience may affect patient satisfaction These would have been controlled if subjects had been randomly allocated between a control and an experimental group. What about other factors that could occur whilst the intervention is in progress? Satisfaction with timed district nursing may be affected by the personality of the nurses rather than the timing of the visit. This is where control of variables through selection of subjects and random allocation becomes so important. The researcher would have to ensure that the same district nurses provided care to both groups. One might try to address this within a pre-test/post-test design by ensuring that the same district nurse visited throughout the intervention. However, that nurse would at some point need some time off and so another nurse might have to be used which could influence patient satisfaction. This means that a pre-test/post-test design is not the best design to use in this situation.

ACTIVITY 16 ALLOW **15** MINUTES

Read the case study below and then answer the questions that follow.

Pre-test/post-test design without controls

Dave is a consultant stoma-care nurse. His role includes teaching sessions to student nurses and he has designed a new, updated education programme for qualified health professionals. The programme is designed to enhance both the knowledge and attitudes of health professionals about stoma care.

The course leader informs Dave that there is little time in the curriculum and that only one group are at the stage in their education where this input is required.

Dave therefore evaluates his programme by administering a pre-test (testing both knowledge and attitudes) before the course (intervention) and then administers the same test (post-test) after the course. If scores on both attitudes and knowledge are higher at the end than the beginning , Dave will assume that his course was successful in teaching participants about stoma care.

1   What factors (extraneous variables), other than the programme itself, could account for the increase in knowledge gained at the end of the programme?

2   In what way could these extraneous factors have been controlled by using an experimental, rather than a quasi-experimental design?

3   Why would Dave have used the same test at the end of the course as the one he used at the beginning?

Commentary

1   Extraneous factors that could account for the increase in knowledge include the possibility that the participants were exposed to some other information during the intervention, such as a magazine article in the *Nursing Times*, which also influenced their knowledge and attitudes.

2   The extraneous variables could have been controlled if Dave had been able to use a control group. Because subjects would be randomly allocated between the intervention group and a control group, both of these groups would be equally likely to have seen the magazine article. Therefore, any differences between the groups at post-test could be assumed to result from the course.

3   Dave would have used the same test at the end of the course as the one he used at the beginning so that he could be sure he was testing the same knowledge and attitude characteristics on each occasion. It would be pointless establishing a baseline measurement of one set of characteristics if a different set was then tested at the end. Dave wouldn't be able to assess whether and how the participants' knowledge had increased.

We can build up our diagram of research methodology again by inserting a pre-test/post-test design without a control group. Our revised diagram appears in *Figure 4* . For ease of reference, only the lower half of the original diagram is reproduced.

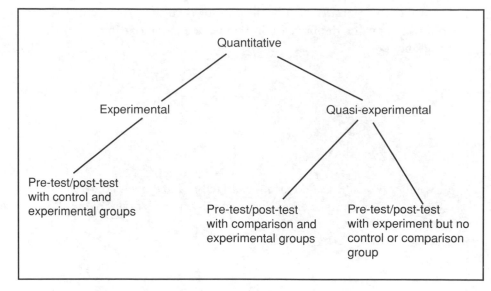

Figure 4: Experimental and quasi-experimental designs

As our research becomes less controlled we can be less certain that what we *think* is causing the change is actually doing so. Clearly, a pre-test/post-test design without either a control or comparison group will be less convincing than if such groups were used. However, pre-test/post-test designs are a better alternative to post-test only designs which we will discuss next.

Post-test only designs

In situations in which it is not possible to use a pre test/post-test design, a post-test only design can be used. Clearly, if you use this design you will not be able to compare the findings of your post-test with the pre-test. A control group or comparison group is vital in this situation to ensure that the findings are credible.

The notation for a comparison group post-test only is as follows:

experimental group   X   0

comparison group   0

Both groups are given a post-test (**0**), but only the experimental group has been given the new programme (**X**).

Remember, if you are using either an experimental or quasi-experimental design some type of comparison is *essential* in order to demonstrate that the change in the relevant characteristics (the independent variable) was in fact due to the intervention.

We will now discuss one final quasi-experimental design, known as a 'time series design' which can be used with one group over a period of time.

Time series design

Skill mix: *A mix of staff (professional and non-professional) to meet standards, outcomes and client expectations fostered by the organisation.*

The following example will serve to explain why time series designs are used.

Imagine that you are a district nurse in a health trust in the north of England which has decided to be the first trust in the region to implement **skill mix** in district nursing. A nurse researcher wishes to assess the effects of skill mix on staff morale as reflected in staff turnover, sickness and number of promotions. The only other trust to have implemented skill mix is in the south east of England and is insufficiently similar (due to the age and experience of the staff and different working patterns) to form a comparison group.

One way to assess the effects would be to administer a pre-test (say in January) and a post-test (in July) which would enable the researcher to see whether there were any differences in the numbers of sickness absences, staff turnover and promotions during the six-month period after the implementation of skill mix.

This sounds fine initially, but what if this six-month period is abnormal in some way – for example a flu epidemic causes an unusually high incidence of sickness? We could not then presume that low morale due to skill mix was responsible for high sickness levels. Furthermore, other policies implemented during the study period, such as GP fundholding, could also be responsible for low morale. Equally, high staff turnover might not be due to low morale, but because a neighbouring trust is offering child-care facilities or a higher salary.

One way of obtaining more reliable results in this kind of situation is to use a 'time series design'. Data is collected at intervals *before* and *after* the programme – thus giving an extended time span of observation and greater control over variables. This is indicated by the following notation:

$$01 \quad 02 \quad 03 \quad 04 \quad X \quad 05 \quad 06 \quad 07 \quad 08$$

Eight different observations are made, four of which (01 02 03 04) are made at specified intervals before the intervention (X) and four (05 06 07 08) *after* the intervention.

In this design, measurements are taken at regular intervals, beginning before the programme is implemented and ending after the programme is concluded. The value of regular testing is in the trends indicated in the results. A gradual increase in sickness levels *throughout* the study period, combined with gradual increases in staff turnover and decreases in staff promotion may be indicative of low morale. Equally, a 'blip' in the results during a particular month may have a specific cause, like a flu epidemic.

We can now return to our diagram for the last time to insert the designs we have recently discussed. A revised version of the diagram is shown in *Figure 5*.

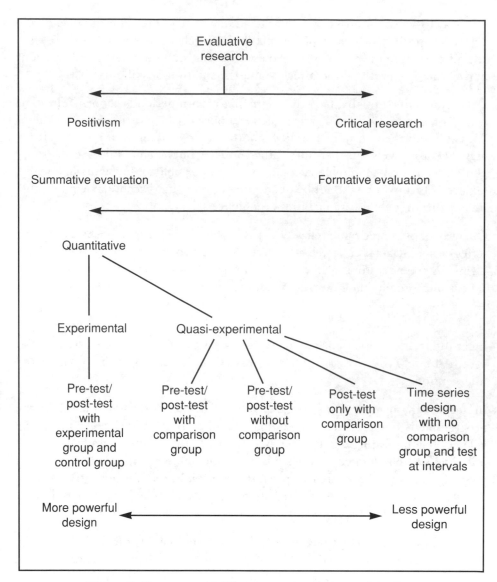

Figure 5: The power of different quasi-experimental designs

Threats to validity in quasi-experimental research

We will now consider some of the threats to internal validity that may lead us to question the 'truth' value of the results obtained from quasi-experimental research. Such factors include:

- **History.** This refers to events external to the treatment that happen at the same time and which could affect the results. GP fundholding, if implemented at the same time as skill mix, could be an extraneous variable which may 'confound' (cause confusion in) the results. In a true experiment (that is, not a quasi-experimental one) in which subjects are randomly allocated to the two groups, GP fundholding would be just as likely to affect the control group as the experimental group. Any differences between the groups could then be assumed to be due to the implementation of skill mix.

- **Selection.** Because the groups are not randomly selected they may be different in some way. The post-test results may therefore reflect the differences in the two groups rather than the treatment. User satisfaction with service provision is an example of this. One group might be comprised of young people who have different expectations to those of the old people in the other group.

- **Maturation**. This refers to processes occurring in the subjects during the course of study as a result of time rather than the intervention. For example, human beings develop and grow regardless of intervention and this means that the natural healing process would ensure that wounds might heal to some extent without specific intervention. The healing of wounds could be a natural process rather than the result of the intervention.

- **Testing**. This refers to the effects of the pre-test on the post-test. This is particularly relevant in the measurement of attitudes. For example, using a pre-test to measure students' attitudes towards AIDS prior to attendance on an AIDS-awareness course may sensitise subjects to the type of attitudes they should have. The results of the post-test may therefore reflect changes resulting from the pre-test as much as from the intervention (the course).

- **Mortality**. This refers to loss of subjects during the course of the study so that those who remain to complete post-test questionnaires may be different in some way. For example, subjects who are dissatisfied may have opted out of the programme so that only satisfied subjects remain. If the intention of the study is to measure satisfaction levels, then clearly the results would be biased.

| ACTIVITY 17 | ALLOW 30 MINUTES |

Read the four case studies below and then complete the table indicating the characteristics of each.

Case Study 1

Linda is a care assistant in a home for older people. As part of a GNVQ course she has read an article discussing the value of staff accompanying confused residents when they wander. The article suggested that the common practice of restraining residents by locking doors causes further disorientation so that residents wander more inside the building and become more disorientated. Accompanying residents outside the building in order to allow them to explore their surroundings had been found to decrease their wandering around the inside of the building (which often caused them to become distressed).

Linda asks the officer in charge for permission to accompany two confused residents throughout their period of wandering, for one week during each of her shifts. Before she starts the intervention she asks each member of staff to document the number and length of times each of the two residents wanders during a three-day period. She then implements her intervention. At the end of the one-week period, members of staff repeat the measurements that were made before the intervention. The frequency and duration of wandering before and after the intervention is then compared.

Case Study 2

Jackie is a health visitor who is interested in reducing the incidence of head injuries to children under five years in her area. She designs a leaflet informing parents about the frequency of head injuries in children and how they can be prevented. She then distributes the leaflets to parents on her caseload over a six-month period. She compares the incidence of head injuries in her area with the district as a whole by examining accident and emergency department (A and E) records for the six month period. This information will give her:

- the number of children with head injuries requiring A and E attendance both before and after the intervention in her area

- the number of children with head injuries requiring A and E attendance in other areas throughout the district during the period of study.

Case Study 3

John is a learning disability nurse working with clients who exhibit challenging behaviour. He has read about a new method of teaching people more social behaviours called 'gentle teaching'. This method opposes the traditional belief that behaviour can be modified by a series of rewards and reinforcements which 'shape' the desirable behaviour. Rather, gentle teaching suggests that clients will slowly alter their behaviour through the use of very gentle client-centred methods. John decides to test the hypothesis that 'gentle teaching' is more effective in reducing challenging behaviour than behaviour modification.

He negotiates with a manager of a community group home for people with learning disabilities to randomly allocate the residents into two groups, one of which will receive gentle teaching and the other behaviour modification. Before he begins the programme he asks staff to record all evidence of challenging behaviour in residents, including frequency, intensity and duration. At the end of the programme the same measurements are taken and compared with those taken before the programme. The incidence of challenging behaviour between the two groups is then compared.

Case Study 4

Sally is a midwifery tutor who wishes to run a series of lectures for student midwives in their final year of training on 'partnership and empowerment'. She wants to evaluate the success of her lectures in enhancing positive attitudes towards partnership and empowerment in students. She is also interested in whether these attitudes are maintained over a lengthy period of time following qualification.

She randomly allocates students to two groups, one of which receives her lectures and another which has its usual lectures. Before commencing the lectures she administers an attitude test to both groups. Immediately following the series of lectures she administers the same attitude questionnaire to both groups. In order to ascertain the differences in attitude between the two groups, she administers the same test after a six-month period (immediately following qualification) and then again after a twelve-month period. At each stage of this process she compares the results of both groups.

	Type of research: experimental or quasi-experimental	Type of design	Threats to validity
Case Study 1			
Case Study 2			
Case Study 3			
Case Study 4			

Commentary

The answers to this activity are presented in the table below.

	Type of research: experimental or quasi-experimental	Type of design	Threats to validity
Case Study 1	quasi-experimental	pre-test/post-test without controls	history – other factors could account for the change, e.g. visit from family, staff on duty
Case Study 2	quasi-experimental	pre-test/post-test with comparison group	selection – groups may be different, e.g. social class, age of parents, type of housing
Case Study 3	experimental	pre-test/post-test with control group	history – some residents may exhibit less challenging behaviour when certain staff are on duty
Case Study 4	experimental	time-series design with control group	history – other factors, e.g. reading about empowerment could account for the results maturity – some students may change naturally and their attitudes may change as a consequence testing – the pre-test may sensitise the groups to the attitudes that they should hold mortality – over such a lengthy period some students may have left, resulting in the remaining ones having certain characteristics.

Summary

1 During this session we have made considerable progress in our discussion and application of evaluative research. We have introduced the first decision you will need to make as an evaluative researcher – whether to use a summative or formative research design.

2 We have identified several designs appropriate to these two approaches which we then divided further into experimental and quasi-experimental designs. We have discussed the strengths and weaknesses of these two major designs and considered them in relation to the black box.

3 We considered the use of specific forms of notation in experimental and quasi-experimental research designs and related these to pre- and post-test situations.

4 We discussed the notion of validity, particularly some of the threats to internal validity in quasi-experimental research. In so doing it is important to recognise that truth may be compromised in different ways.

Before you move on to Session Four, check that you have achieved the objectives given at the beginning of this session and, if not, review the appropriate sections.

Approaches to evaluative research

Introduction

This session is designed to increase your confidence in evaluating the services you deliver by guiding you through the important decisions you need to make in evaluative research. You will then be able to select an appropriate research design to meet the needs of any people who have a stake in your research, such as those who fund your research and people who have a vested interest in the research findings.

Session objectives

When you have completed this session you should be able to:

- describe the advantages and disadvantages of the following approaches to evaluative research:

  the experimental

  the goal-orientated

  the decision-focused

  the user-orientated

  the responsive.

- describe why the responsive approach is an example of critical research methodology.

1: Choosing an approach

Your choice of approach will depend on what you are evaluating and your relationship with the decision-makers as well as the service users. Some types of service will require an experimental approach as discussed in Session Three, for example those in which effectiveness is measured using scientific measurements like blood pressure recordings or blood tests. Other services would need to be evaluated using more qualitative methods. This can be described as a 'responsive' approach to evaluation – for example, naturalistic observation methods could be used to measure the effectiveness of a programme of reminiscence therapy sessions in which older people are encouraged to recall and talk about past events. These are two of the five approaches possible in evaluative research discussed by Stecher and Davis (1987):

- experimental

- goal-orientated

- decision-focused

- user-orientated

- responsive.

We will now look at each of these in turn.

The experimental approach

We discussed experimental methods in some detail in Session Two and in more depth in Session Three. The section in Session Three entitled 'Quasi-experimental research' lists the three characteristics of a true experiment. The following activity will serve as a reminder of the main characteristics of the experimental approach.

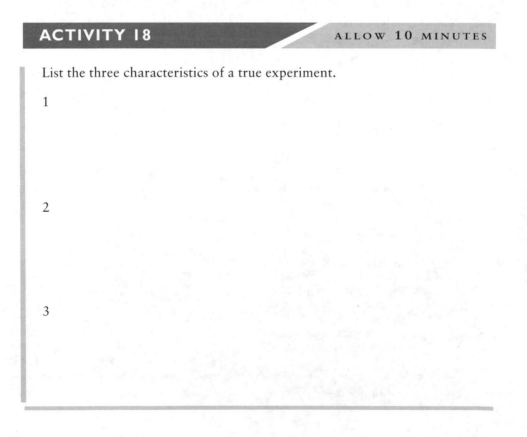

ACTIVITY 18　　　　　ALLOW **10** MINUTES

List the three characteristics of a true experiment.

1

2

3

Commentary

The three characteristics of the experimental approach are:

1 *random* allocation of subjects to two groups

2 *control* of variables

3 *manipulation* of the experiment by the researcher.

The main strengths of the experimental approach are that it is:

- more objective because it is not open to the interpretation of the researcher

- more generalisable to other populations because the findings are valid and reliable

- more credible because of the above.

The weaknesses of this approach are that:

- it is difficult to control variables in the real world. The researcher is often unable to use laboratory conditions for experiments on human subjects and the fact that people will inevitably be exposed to other lifestyle factors often contaminates the research findings

- due to the attempt to control variables, it is insensitive to the complexities of human interaction that could be elicited through, for example, interviews

- it reduces the complexities of human interaction to characteristics that can be scientifically tested, measured and counted. Rather than understanding the deep concerns of subjects, the researcher concentrates on small elements of behaviour that can be counted or measured in some way.

Before we move on to the second approach to evaluation we will return briefly to our earlier discussions of formative and summative evaluation and critical research methodology and revise how experimental methods can be applied to these approaches in the following activity.

ACTIVITY 19   ALLOW 15 MINUTES

1 Which kind of evaluation can the experimental method be used in – formative or summative?

2 Is the experimental approach an example of critical research methodology? Give reasons for your answer.

Commentary

1 This type of research is more likely to be used as summative evaluation because the experimental evaluator is only interested in inputs and outputs. This means controlling the experiment (inputs) and analysing the results (outputs). Due to the need for tight controls and strict measurements, it is often carried out by professional researchers or even teams of researchers – which also makes it more typical of summative evaluation. The experimental researcher would be unlikely to encourage interference from the decision-makers during the evaluation because this could contaminate the findings. The findings would only be written up and reported at the end of the evaluation rather than at various stages of the research as is the case in formative evaluation.

2 The distance between the researcher and the service user in experimental research prevents the experimental approach from being critical research methodology. The necessity for the researcher to maintain controlled conditions will render him or her uninterested in acting as an advocate for, or in empowering, the subjects of the experiment. Clearly, to become emotionally involved to this extent would threaten the objective nature of experimental research and would therefore reduce its credibility. As you will recall from Session One, critical research methodology involves the key characteristics of advocacy, activism, empowerment and emancipation. These characteristics require that the researcher becomes actively involved with the needs of the subjects of the study rather than act as a detached observer of the variables under study. The lack of interest in what is happening during the research (the contents of the black box) makes the experimental approach an example of summative evaluation and not an example of critical research methodology.

In the continuum of approaches to evaluation identified by Stecher and Davis (1987) the experimental approach is the most scientific. It requires the researcher to be active in manipulating and gaining control of the experiment by assigning subjects to groups and controlling unwanted influences. Despite this activity on the part of the researcher, he or she must also distance him or herself from the subjects so that objectivity can be maintained.

A slightly less scientific approach to evaluative research is the goal-orientated approach, which we will discuss next.

The goal-orientated approach

The goal-orientated approach is, as its name suggests, interested in evaluating *whether* and *the extent to which* the programme has been successful in achieving its *goals*. For this reason it is first necessary to identify the goals of the programme and the activities designed to achieve them.

According to Stecher and Davis the purpose of the goal-orientated approach is to:

● measure the attainment of the programme's goals

● encourage those developing research to clarify objectives in measurable terms

● clarify implementation plans.

The programme objectives therefore need to be stated in a way that can subsequently be measured by the researcher. The implementation of the programme also needs to be clear so that the researcher knows precisely what it is that is to be evaluated. The following case study shows an example of a goal-orientated approach.

A goal-orientated approach

Julie is a ward sister on a children's ward. The paediatrician is interested in a new, radical system of diagnosing 'Munchausen syndrome by proxy' (a condition in which parents harm their children by making them ill). The system involves the use of covert video surveillance of parents and their children whilst in hospital in order to detect the condition. Julie thinks this system is unethical and only agrees to its implementation on condition that it can be evaluated in order to demonstrate that it is a suitable method of diagnosing this condition. She insists that the goals of the programme must be clearly specified and measured. The goals are stated as being to:

- identify parents who need assistance with parenting skills

- provide support and counselling to such parents

- detect parents who are harming their children

- protect children at risk of harm or neglect by their parents

- diagnose 'Munchausen syndrome by proxy'.

Julie uses the following resources to implement the programme:

- a surveillance camera

- a room with a one-way mirror through which the surveillance takes place

- a member of staff to observe the video screen continually

- a training programme for staff involved in the programme

- a support service for parents

- a system of liaison with the social services department and the police service.

This case study demonstrates how a programme in which goals are clearly specified helps the programme developer plan its implementation, including planning the resources which will be needed. The evaluative researcher would be able to measure the effectiveness of such a programme by establishing the extent to which each objective has been achieved. The evaluator would also need to decide which measurement tools would be required to measure the achievement of each objective. We will return to this issue of selecting measuring tools in Session Five.

The case study also clearly illustrates the strengths of the goal-orientated approach. According to Stecher and Davis these are:

- the logical relationship between the programme objectives and activities occurring within the programme. The covert video surveillance programme, for example, uses specific tools to achieve the goals of the programme, such as video equipment, training of staff and liaison with other services. The logical relationship is evident because the goals of the programme are achieved through the use of the various types of equipment and staff.

- the emphasis on specific elements of the programme that require evaluating. This focuses the concern of the researcher onto the important issues defined by programme developers. The different elements of the surveillance programme are specified in such a way that they could be evaluated separately. For example, staff training would be evaluated separately from the perceptions of the parents about the support they had received.

The weaknesses of this approach are that:

- by focusing on very specific issues the researcher may miss unintended consequences of the programme that are worthy of evaluation. For example, he or she may focus so closely on the specific goals of the programme and the resources required that he or she fails to recognise that the covert surveillance programme is conveying important information about parent/child interactions which have nothing to do with the condition but which could result in anti-social behaviour patterns in the children as they grow up.

- the researcher may overlook important issues associated with the design of the programme due to focusing exclusively on the achievement of objectives. For example, the way this programme is to be conducted could ethically compromise researchers. This issue would need to be addressed before going ahead with the research, as staff would need to be trained specifically to deal with this. If the researcher was very keen on achieving the objectives he or she might ignore this matter.

The researcher will need to work quite closely with programme developers to determine how to evaluate programme objectives, and often the researcher will need to work quite closely with participants such as staff and children. The *psychological distance* between researcher and subjects is, therefore, much smaller than in the experimental approach. The goal-orientated approach is therefore more subjective and less scientific. Furthermore, unlike in the experimental approach, few statistical tests will be used to analyse the data gathered.

ACTIVITY 20　　　　ALLOW 15 MINUTES

1　Do you think the goal-orientated approach could be used in formative or summative evaluation? Give reasons for your answer.

2　Is the goal-orientated approach an example of critical research methodology? Give reasons for your answer.

Commentary

1   The goal-orientated approach is more suited to formative than summative evaluation because the criteria outlined by Thorpe (1988) which we discussed in Session Three are met, namely:

   ● the research would be driven by decision-makers rather than by the preferences of the researcher or the needs of the clients

   ● there would be an element of monitoring involved

   ● there would be constant feedback to decision-makers

   ● the research would probably be carried out by staff and would be reported locally.

2   The goal-orientated approach is not an example of critical research methodology. The researcher does not get sufficiently involved in the lives of the participants to act as an advocate or to empower them to instigate social change. The researcher is focusing exclusively on whether or not the goals of the programme are achieved.

We will now move on to consider the third approach to evaluative research identified by Stecher and Davis – the decision-focused approach.

The decision-focused approach

As its name implies, this approach is concerned with the provision of information to programme managers in order to assist decision-making. The key characteristic of the decision-focused approach is that the researcher consults with key decision-makers at some point during the research because the purpose of the research is to attend to the needs of the decision-makers. Ideally, the decision-orientated evaluator should be involved with the programme during its development stage so that he or she can collaborate with decision-makers in deciding how the programme can be evaluated. If the evaluator is not present during this stage, the decision-makers would themselves decide on how to evaluate the programme. The evaluation task would be given to the researcher once the research design had already been determined.

You may have already realised that decision-focused evaluation is becoming more common in health and social care. Rarely is a new system of delivering care developed without someone asking 'how is this going to be evaluated?' It is this serious consideration of evaluation at the programme development stage that means a decision-focused approach is being used.

The evaluator will need to know:

● the important decision points during the development of the programme

● the kind of information which might illuminate each decision.

Armed with this information the evaluator will be able to design measuring tools to collect the type of data required at the most important times. The following case study illustrates the use of a decision-focused approach.

The decision-focused approach

Morag is a nurse researcher who has been appointed by the ENB to conduct a research project to evaluate the transition of colleges of nursing into existing universities. The ENB has already negotiated with three colleges of nursing to use them for the project. The research is to run alongside the transition of the colleges into the universities so that:

- the ENB, together with college management teams, can decide how the transition can best be evaluated

- any difficulties related to the transition, such as staff development needs, can be identified early so that decision-makers can make any necessary changes promptly

- Morag can be invited to all meetings concerning the transition so that she can be advised of the important developments and can incorporate them into her evaluation plans.

As part of her contract, Morag is required to present a report of her research developments to the ENB every three months. The ENB will then send copies of her reports to each of the colleges of nursing.

The strengths of this approach are that it:

- attends to the specific needs of decision-makers and is driven by decision-makers rather than the researcher. This ensures that the research is supported by those who will provide the funding

- provides influential evaluations at relevant points which are important to the decision-making process.

The weaknesses of this approach are that:

- many important decisions are reached gradually, not at specific points, and the researcher may not therefore be in a position to provide the relevant data at the appropriate time. In fact, many important decisions are often made informally in corridors and on staircases!

- decisions may not always be data-based but may be based on subjective impressions

- the data provided by the researcher may not necessarily provide an accurate picture of the needs of service users because there may be a discrepancy between what the decision-maker wants the researcher to find out, and what service users really need.

ACTIVITY 21　　　　　ALLOW 20 MINUTES

1 Do you think that the decision-focused approach would be used in formative or summative evaluation? Give reasons for your answer.

2 Do you think that the decision-focused approach is an example of critical research methodology? Give reasons for your answer.

Commentary

1 The decision-focused approach could be an example of either formative or summative evaluation, depending on how the research is to be carried out. In the example we have used, a final summative report would be required. However, the frequent contact with decision-makers and the opportunity to impact on the development of the programme during the research, is typical of formative evaluation.

2 The approach is not an example of critical research methodology. Although an evaluator may have the opportunity to activate service users and staff into lobbying decision-makers and politicians to influence policy, he or she will mostly be limited by decision-makers who dictate the type of data to be collected and from whom it is to be collected. The data gathering in critical research methodology must be meaningful for the decision-making process and not just for the evaluator. This fact alone makes the decision-focused approach less appropriate for critical research methodology. Decision-makers may not be interested in the real needs of service users, particularly if these would demand costly resources.

We will now look at an approach which favours service users rather than decision-makers – the 'user-orientated approach'.

The user-orientated approach

Unlike other approaches to evaluation discussed so far, this approach requires the direct involvement of the client throughout. The task of the evaluator is to create a working group of key users. Once the group is formed it:

- designs the evaluation

- decides what measurements will be taken and the instruments to be used

- chooses when measurements will be taken

- selects subjects to be used.

Since the research is set up by users of the service, the needs of the researcher are subordinated to those of the users (although the researcher will have to assist them with the research design and choice of measuring instruments).

The relationship between the researcher and the users could be described as circular. The researcher receives suggestions from users, proposes ideas in response to them and then adapts the evaluation to the needs of the client. Patton (1986) describes this as 'an active, reactive, adaptive approach'. We have illustrated this in Figure 6.

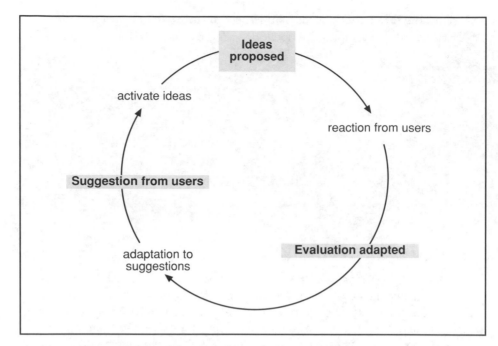

Figure 6: The active, reactive, adaptive approach to evaluation

The following case study illustrates the use of the user-orientated approach.

The user-orientated approach

Mo is a social worker working in an area of high social deprivation. He is involved with a group of local people and community professionals who are setting up a food co-operative for the benefit of the local population. The group has rented a small warehouse in which they will store food and other goods which they buy at cost price from distributors. They will then sell the goods to the local population without making a profit.

Mo has decided that he would like to evaluate the effectiveness of the initiative. He organises a meeting with all those involved in the programme to discuss what elements of the programme they should evaluate and how they should go about it.

The strengths of this approach are that:

● it relies on people who care about the programme. The researcher is likely to gain co-operation from all concerned when collecting data

● there is attention to gathering meaningful information because the information needed is decided upon by the users as well as decision-makers

● it is concerned with ownership of the evaluation. Because both users and decision-makers are involved in the evaluation the findings are more likely to be implemented than left in a dusty file.

The weaknesses of this approach are that:

● it requires a stable user group. If group members change frequently alternative views may result in a lack of consistency in the evaluation

● there may be undue influence from some members. Stronger members of the working group may influence others and this may be detrimental to the evaluation, particularly if this results in an imbalance in participation.

ACTIVITY 22   ALLOW 15 MINUTES

1 Do you think that the user-orientated approach would be used in formative or summative evaluation? Give reasons for your answer.

2 Do you think that the user-orientated approach is an example of critical research methodology? Give reasons for your answer.

Commentary

1 Because the user-orientated approach relies so strongly on the input of users it is more likely to be used in formative evaluation. Far from being carried out by expert researchers, the research is designed by those interested in the programme. Such an approach is:

● inexpensive

● local in orientation

● able to feed the results back into the programme at any stage in the evaluation so that necessary changes can be made to benefit service users.

2 The involvement of users also enables the researcher to activate and empower all those involved in the programme. The researcher is receptive to all suggestions made by the user groups. This means, for example, that employees who may not normally have much say in decision-making are given an opportunity to inform policy. For this reason the user-orientated approach to evaluation is a good example of critical research methodology.

It is clear that the different approaches to evaluative research discussed so far have become increasingly less scientific and less orientated to the desires of the researcher. This is also evident in the final approach to evaluative research discussed by Stecher and Davis (1987) – the responsive approach.

The responsive approach

The responsive approach is so-called because it seeks to respond to issues from the multiple perspectives of programme developers. It is therefore very similar to the user-orientated approach. It attempts to understand multiple viewpoints by listening to the views of all the stakeholders. This approach requires that the researcher use multiple methods of data collection, in particular naturalistic methods such as observation, interviews and conversations. The researcher then interprets the findings using his or her own impressions of the data. This approach, then, requires that the researcher adopt the role of an organisational anthropologist. The following case study illustrates the use of the responsive approach.

The responsive approach

Jane is a health visitor attached to a large general practice. She has identified, through discussion with the GP, that a large number of young women in the practice have visited the GP due to depressive illness. Most of them have young children and live on a new housing estate.

Jane works with Sandra (the practice nurse) to set up a support group for all mothers with children under two years. They decide to facilitate the group until natural leaders emerge who they hope will take over the running of future groups and develop an outreach service to other young mothers who need support.

They decide to evaluate the programme by discussing with the mothers and the GP what they would like to achieve from the programme. An agreement is drawn up stating that if at any time problems arise with the programme, Jane and Sandra will respond to their needs.

Jane and Sandra decide to evaluate the programme using naturalistic methods. They therefore observe events as they occur in the group sessions. They use field notes to write down their observations and take particular note of any changes in members of the group, such as growth in confidence, willingness to participate and taking the lead. They also record conversations they have with participants which could be used as data demonstrating the effectiveness of the programme.

Throughout the process Jane and Sandra share their findings with the participants and the GP, so that any concerns can be responded to at an early stage. Jane's manager is also kept informed of developments because, if successful, the group may be repeated elsewhere.

The strengths of this approach are that:

- it is sensitive to the multiple viewpoints of the different stakeholders – the views of all those involved, including clients and staff, are valued

- it can deal with poorly focused concerns and conflicting views because it is open to events as they occur and no behaviour or event is 'screened out'

- it assists in the understanding of a variety of issues because of the richness of the data.

The weaknesses of this approach are that:

- the very richness of the data makes it difficult to simplify information for decision-making

- it is impossible to act on all views. For example, the views of clients may conflict with those of staff. The researcher can, therefore, *take account* of all views, but may not be able to *act* on all of them.

ACTIVITY 23 — ALLOW 15 MINUTES

1   Do you think that the responsive approach would be used in formative or summative evaluation? Give reasons for your answer.

2   Do you think that the responsive approach is an example of critical research methodology? Give reasons for your answer.

Commentary

1   The responsive approach is more conducive to formative than summative evaluation because the researcher constantly reports their impressionistic interpretation to the stakeholders. The evaluator is more likely to be asking 'how is this going?' and 'how can we improve it?' rather than 'was it worth doing?' and 'should we continue with it?'

2   Whether or not the responsive approach is an example of critical research methodology is a difficult question to answer because the researcher may be responding to the concerns of decision-makers for a large proportion of the evaluation, rather than to those of service users. If, however, the researcher uses his or her position to act as an advocate for clients or to activate them to state how they feel their service should be improved, then the evaluation is moving more towards critical research methodology.

Whether or not the evaluator is using a user-orientated approach would depend on the methodology used. For example, naturalistic observation is more likely to be used in the responsive approach than in the user-orientated approach. The researcher using the responsive approach is responsive to the multiple perspectives of different stakeholders rather than just to the users and so needs to 'juggle' the needs of the various people involved in the programme. This may result in the researcher attending to the needs of the decision-makers rather than the service users so that critical research methodology would not be being used.

ACTIVITY 24

In order to ensure you understand the five approaches to evaluation, complete the missing names of the relevant research approaches in the far left-hand column of the table below.

Approach	Role of researcher	Formative/ summative	Critical research method
	Random allocation Control of variables	Summative	No
	Have programme objectives been achieved?	Probably formative Could be summative	No
	Work with decision-makers to decide on evaluation during development and implementation	Formative	No
	Develop working group of users to design evaluation	Formative	Yes, if interest in users' needs leads to close involvement of researcher in clients' lives with aim of bringing about social change
	Responds to needs of various stakeholders in designing research	Formative	Need to respond to needs of different stakeholders could create conflict. Only critical if needs of users take priority and researcher able to engage in social change

Commentary

Your completed box should look like the table below.

Approach	Role of researcher	Formative/ summative	Critical research method
Experimental	Random allocation Control of variables	Summative	No
Goal-orientated	Have programme objectives been achieved?	Probably formative Could be summative	No
Decision-focused	Work with decision-makers to decide on evaluation during development and implementation	Formative	No
User-orientated	Develop working group of users to design evaluation	Formative	Yes, if interest in users' needs leads to close involvement of researcher in clients' lives with aim of bringing about social change
Responsive	Responds to needs of various stakeholders in designing research	Formative	Need to respond to needs of different stakeholders could create conflict. Only critical if needs of users take priority and researcher able to engage in social change

2: Assessing the value of the various approaches

We can now see that choosing an approach to evaluative research is quite a complex affair. How do we make decisions about which approach to use? First, the *methodology* in evaluative research is less important than the *issues concerning the stakeholders* in the programme. Therefore, before you select an approach you need to decide whose needs you are addressing. For example, are you trying to help decision-makers or the users of your service? The needs of each may require very different approaches to data collection. We will discuss this in more detail in the next session.

Once you have decided whose needs you are serving you need to be aware of any limitations this may have for your methodology. Early evaluation methods used in the 1920s and 1930s, such as the experimental approach, raise important ethical issues. Is it justified, for example, to deny some people a beneficial programme in order to fulfil the randomisation requirement of experimental research? Unlike more recent evaluators, early programme evaluators distanced themselves from the political and ethical dimensions of their work intentionally in order to remain objective and scientific.

More recently, during the 1980s and 1990s, evaluators have recognised their importance in influencing the decision-making process. By the very nature of evaluation the researcher is engaged in a political activity because research findings will have an effect on the provision of services. If, as a programme evaluator, you demonstrate that a programme is meeting its goals, then there will be no need for the organisation running the programme to increase the provision. Far from attempting to remain neutral and objective, the contemporary evaluator is likely to want to get involved in the programme he or she is researching because he or she is involved with and concerned about the service users.

Decision-focused, user-orientated and responsive approaches also have implications for the researcher in relation to influencing political decisions. Do you wish to respond to the needs of distant decision-makers or are you more concerned with local people who have a stake in the programme? These could include managers, staff and users. Stake (1978) argues that attention to local needs is more responsive and will produce a richer experiential understanding than simply responding to the needs of decision-makers.

Critics of the goal-orientated approach such as Scriven (1967) suggest that social programmes should be evaluated according to the merit and worth of their *actual* effects, independent of their *intended* effects. Scriven (1973) developed this argument into a recommendation for a 'goal-free' approach as opposed to a 'goal-orientated'one. He suggested that it is more important to uncover whether or not a programme meets the needs of its users than to find out whether it meets its goals. This suggests that the goals of the programme may be inappropriate and guided by organisational and political ends rather than the needs of consumers. Polit and Hungler (1987) also point out that establishing goals may be difficult anyway, because programme goals are often multiple and diffuse. Some elements of a programme might be successful where others were not, so the researcher would not be able to say whether the programme as a whole had succeeded.

The responsive approach, as we have already discussed, moves us towards using qualitative methods of collecting data. Greene (1994) particularly favours qualitative methods for evaluative research. She says that qualitative researchers should be more concerned with the *context* of their findings, rather than with how generalisable they are to other populations. This means that the researcher is concerned with whether the findings are an accurate depiction of the context in which they occured – are they in fact *true?* For Greene (1994), qualitative programme evaluators, rather than distancing themselves from the study as the early evaluators did, actually 'celebrate' their presence by using their own interpretation of events to enhance their understanding. If you decide to get involved with participants to this extent you will be using a critical research approach to evaluation.

Before we conclude this session, one final activity will serve to illustrate a typical approach to evaluative research used in the 1990s.

ACTIVITY 25   ALLOW 15 MINUTES

Imagine that you are the officer in charge of a social services hostel for people with learning disabilities. The social services department you work for has commissioned a programme evaluator to evaluate the services provided for people with learning disabilities throughout the district. Because your hostel has been selected as part of a sample, you and your team are the target group for the collection of data. The stakeholders in the programme are:

- the residents

- the social services department

- you and your staff.

Write down some thoughts on the following questions.

1   Would you feel that your own personal concerns about service provision should be taken into account and why?

2   How would you feel about the researcher interviewing you about your work with the residents?

3   Would it be acceptable, instead, for the researcher to interview the residents without your knowledge (because they might give more honest answers this way) and then feed back the findings directly to your employer?

Commentary

1   You would probably feel that you would like your own personal concerns about service provision to be taken into account because, since you work closely with residents, you may well have more insight into their needs than either the decision maker or a researcher.

2   You might feel that you would like to discuss the work you do with a researcher because you are confident that you provide a high-quality service. On the other hand, you might feel too busy working with residents

to spend time discussing what you do. Furthermore, you might feel that a researcher may be unnecessarily critical of your work because he or she has insufficient knowledge to understand what you do.

3   You might feel quite comfortable with the researcher interviewing your residents without your knowledge if you are confident that they would speak highly of the service you provide. However, you might feel that various constraints such as shortage of staff make it impossible to provide the kind of service you would like to provide, and that any adverse comments might reflect badly on you as a practitioner rather than on the service as a whole. You would probably want to know what the researcher says to your employers in this case.

The activity illustrates how contemporary evaluation methods such as responsive evaluation, particularly using qualitative methods, can be potentially threatening to stakeholders. Evaluators therefore need to use tact and diplomacy throughout the data-gathering process. The activity also shows how useful responsive evaluation can be in addressing the needs of different people involved in the delivery of services. For example, by asking for your views as well as the views of residents and managers, the researcher could gain a fuller picture of what was happening and both you and your residents might thereby influence the future development of the service.

According to Stake (1991) improvement in service provision is more likely if local concerns (the concerns of those who are delivering the service) rather than remote concerns are addressed. For example, senior managers might decide that the same level of service could be provided with fewer staff, thus saving money which could be used to provide services elsewhere. This would result in a change in service provision, but probably for the worse because the remote managers might be unaware of local needs. The activity shows one way of addressing local concerns including those of both staff and residents because the researcher uses a single team of people (a discrete group in a small hostel) as the source of data. This is often referred to as the 'case study method' because it allows the researcher to focus on local areas of concern (a case) rather than on the larger groups typical of surveys.

Figure 7 shows the interrelationships between the research approaches that we have discussed so far.

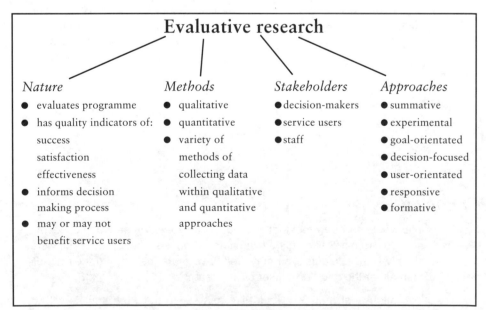

Figure 7: Extended version of *Figure 1* showing the different approaches to evaluative research

Summary

1 The choice of approach to evaluative research has been considered, bearing in mind the nature of services to be evaluated.

2 Five major approaches to evaluative research have been discussed, each of which can be applied successfully to health and social care situations.

3 The strengths and weaknesses of each approach are categorised within a formative and/or summative framework.

4 We have traced the changes in approach to evaluation research from quantitative experimental design to the more responsive, qualitative research approach.

5 The value of each approach has been considered in the light of modern health and social care services.

Before you move on to Session Five, check that you have achieved the objectives given at the beginning of this session and, if not, review the appropriate sections.

Collecting and analysing data for evaluative research

Introduction

The first four sessions of this unit have progressed from looking at the purpose of evaluative research to describing the different approaches and research designs used. We will now look at how the data for an evaluative research study is collected.

This session will take you through the process of deciding upon:

- the setting for your research study

- who to collect data from

- how to get access to those providing data

- what type of data is needed and how to collect it

- how to analyse the data.

We will discuss both qualitative and quantitative methods of collecting and analysing data and will apply our data-collection methods to the five approaches to evaluative research discussed in Session Four.

Session objectives

When you have completed this session you should be able to:

- plan how to gain access to relevant settings for data collection purposes

- select and justify your choice of sampling frame for data collection

- design questionnaires and interview schedules appropriately

- recall how to use descriptive and inferential statistics to analyse survey data from evaluative research

- recall how to use qualitative data analysis to analyse open-ended responses and observations derived from evaluative research.

1: Selecting a research setting

Now that you have some appreciation of how to design an evaluative research study we need to discuss the collection of data. First, you need to establish which of the five approaches you intend to use. You will recall that the five approaches are:

- experimental

- goal-orientated

- decision-focused

- user-orientated

- responsive.

You will also need to decide whether you intend to use a formative or a summative approach.

Target group: *A representative group of people identified as having the necessary characteristics matching the research design.*

You will then need to select the setting which will be the focus of your study. In many cases this will be your own work environment. However, if you were a professional researcher you might be entering an unfamiliar environment and would therefore need to find out how to gain access to your **target group** of respondents, or to records and other documents which would be the basis of your data. Second, you will need to decide which people within the setting you would like to be the target group for your data collection. You might wish to use the entire population of people in the setting or you might wish to select a sample. Third, you will need to decide what type of information (data) you need from your respondents and how to collect it. Finally, you will need to analyse your data.

You should obviously choose a setting that is most likely to provide you with findings that reflect the 'true' nature of the programme in question. You may need to use only one setting, for example if you are using a case study method, or you may need to use two settings, one as a control group and another as an experimental group.

ACTIVITY 26	ALLOW **20** MINUTES

Read the following case study and then answer the questions below.

Evaluative research

Cynthia is a nursery nurse in a day nursery in an inner-city area. The nursery only allows children to attend if they will be staying from 8 am right through to 5 pm. Cynthia has noticed recently that this does not meet the needs of many of the parents who are increasingly working part-time. Cynthia persuades the officer in charge to allow her to introduce three different modes of attendance: all day, 8 am to 12.30 pm and 12.30 to 5 pm. Parents will then be able to decide which mode is most appropriate for them. Cynthia is allowed to introduce the programme provided that if it proves unacceptable to parents it can be discontinued at any stage.

Cynthia states that the objectives of this system are to:

- create more flexibility for parents

- reduce the need for children to spend unnecessary time in the nursery

- create places for more children

- reduce the waiting list

- prevent parents working part-time from being penalised by having to use full-time day-nursery care.

Cynthia monitors each of the objectives over a six-month period to see whether the new system is effective. She does this by sending a questionnaire to all parents to see how satisfied they are with the new system. She also interviews each member of staff to find out what effect the new system has had on their working practices.

Cynthia agrees with the officer in charge that changes that need to be made to the programme as a result of Cynthia's findings, will be made at any stage rather than waiting until the end of the study period.

1   Which of the five approaches to evaluative research is used in this case study? Give reasons for your answer.

2   Is this an example of formative or summative evaluation? Give reasons for your answer.

Commentary

1   The specification of goals (objectives) at the early stage of the research makes the case study typical of a goal-orientated approach. However, because Cynthia attempts to be responsive to the needs of stakeholders by interviewing staff about their views and eliciting the views of parents you might have thought this was an example of responsive research. Nevertheless, as the main emphasis is on the achievement of goals this approach is goal-orientated. The use of questionnaires to establish satisfaction is also more typical of a goal-orientated approach than a responsive approach.

2   Cynthia's research is an example of formative evaluation because:

● she is conducting it herself rather than relying on a team of experts

● it is relatively cheap to carry out because she is collecting information as part of her job

● she is using the research to monitor progress rather than to produce a final research report

● she is prepared to make changes to the programme at any stage, if necessary, rather than wait until the end of the study period.

During this session you are going to design your own evaluative research project and the following activity is the start of this process.

ACTIVITY 27   ALLOW 30 MINUTES

1   Decide on an area relevant to your practice that you would like to evaluate. You may wish to focus on user satisfaction with services, for example, or you may wish to evaluate a recent initiative that has been developed in your area. It would not need to be a large initiative – a small education programme, or a new wound-dressing technique would be sufficient. Write your choice here.

2   State whether a formative or summative evaluation would be most appropriate. Give reasons for your answer.

3   State which of the five approaches to evaluative research you will use.

4   State where you would like to carry out your research. For example, will it be carried out in your own workplace or using your own case load, in a hospital ward, a community, a hostel or a different organisation?

Commentary

Your answers to this activity will obviously be very specific to your area of practice and so you should check them with other students, tutors or a mentor.

Your choice of settings will be determined by the topic chosen and the approach to evaluative research that you have chosen to adopt. If you wish to use a user-orientated or a responsive approach, for example, a small case study with relatively few respondents (such as a ward or department or a health centre) would be quite acceptable.

A goal-orientated approach or decision-focused approach, on the other hand, would require larger sample sizes, because you may need to send questionnaires to a representative sample of the population you are concerned with.

The experimental approach and the quasi-experimental approach in which a comparison group is used differ from the other approaches in that you would need two separate groups from which you would expect to manipulate variables. You may wish to carry out your research in your own work environment or you may wish to access a similar work base. Either of these would be acceptable.

An example of a possible research project is given below.

1   As a community psychiatric nurse (CPN) you wish to evaluate the effectiveness of a programme to support families when a relative with schizophrenia has been discharged home. Evidence suggests that families

in which there is a high degree of 'expressed emotion' may have a detrimental effect on family members suffering from schizophrenia (Bradshaw and Everitt, 1995). You might decide to use family assessment tools such as the Relative Assessment Interview (Barrowclough and Tarrier, 1992) and the Knowledge about Schizophrenia Interview (Barrowclough and Tarrier, 1987) to assess the needs of families in order to set behavioural goals for the patient and the steps needed to achieve them. You could choose to evaluate the effectiveness of these assessment tools in helping you to support families.

2   This would be a formative evaluation because you would be conducting it yourself as a small-scale project and using it to monitor your support of families during your normal working practice.

3   You could use an experimental approach, by randomly allocating families to an 'intervention' (support) group and a control group who would receive the normal CPN service. You could then measure both groups before and after the programme by using a questionnaire indicating family stressors and methods of coping with them.

Alternatively, you could use a goal-orientated approach by clearly specifying the goals of your support programme and then measuring each one of them to see if it has been achieved.

You could also employ a user-orientated approach by contacting key users and other interested people, such as voluntary workers and social workers, and discussing with them how to evaluate the service in a manner which is appropriate to all concerned.

Finally, you could use a responsive approach by observing family interactions as they occur in their natural setting and conversing with families to find out how useful they have found the support they have received.

4   In this situation you would probably carry out the research using families in your own caseload. However, before you started the research, you would need to gain permission from your manager, as well as the local ethics committee, even though you are conducting the research as part of your normal working practice.

2: Gaining access to a research setting

Once you have decided upon the nature of your research, the target group for your data collection and your setting, you can think about gaining access to your chosen setting. This is an important part of the research process which needs careful thought. If you do not use tact and diplomacy and follow any necessary protocols you will not gain the co-operation of people who control access.

It is easy to assume that your wish to collect data will not intrude on the work situation or impose upon staff or clients, and that gaining access is a perfectly reasonable thing to expect from managers. However, the reality of research can be very different. Managers, like any health professional, have a responsibility to safeguard the interests of patients and clients. This means that they will need to be absolutely satisfied that your research is not going to inconvenience service users or staff any more than is necessary. They will also want to be assured that your research is going to be of some benefit to service users rather than merely serving your interests as a researcher.

As discussed in the introductory unit of this series, you need to ask the following of your proposed research.

1 Does it pass the 'so what?' test for research? This means, according to Clark (1987), that it should:

- be relevant to patient/client care, and have the potential to improve client care

- yield results that are of practical value and/or theoretical significance, contributing to the existing body of scientific knowledge

- be useful to other nurses (or other professionals) as well as yourself.

2 Are there any ethical implications? (See the Ethics section in Session Two of the introductory unit.)

Once you have satisfied yourself that your evaluation is of some benefit to users and that it is ethically sound, you should approach the person in charge of the organisation to ask if access may be arranged. You will need to do this in writing, stating the precise nature and purpose of your research. You will need to say:

- what you would like to do

- why you would like to do it

- the benefits it would have for the organisation and the users

- briefly how you intend to collect data.

Managers would probably feel differently about you sending a one-page questionnaire to users, or conducting a 30-minute interview of a small sample, to you using participant observation and 'shadowing' different staff through each shift.

It is important that you think all of these issues through carefully before contacting the person in charge of the organisation. This will help to create the impression of an efficient and organised researcher who is going to create minimal disruption to the organisation. This information will also be required when you seek ethical approval – which you will need to do whenever you intend to obtain information from any kind of service users.

Once you have gained permission to conduct your research you will then proceed to the ethical approval stage. You will need to find out how often local ethics committees meet. This may vary from monthly to three-monthly, or even less frequently. You therefore need to build time for ethical approval into the time-scale for your research. The person who gives you permission to undertake the study (normally the person in charge of the organisation) will be a good place to start in ascertaining the procedure for ethical approval.

If you are registered as a student with a university or another educational institution, the institution may also have an ethics committee from which you will need approval as well.

ACTIVITY 28

1 Find out who you need to contact for permission to gain access to the organisation in which you would like to carry out your research.

2 Draft a letter to the person concerned requesting permission to conduct your research. Remember to include the level of detail indicated earlier.

3 Find out the protocol for gaining ethical approval and write brief notes below as a reminder to yourself.

Commentary

Because of the personal nature of this activity specific advice would be inappropriate. However, it would be useful at this point to share your findings with other students, a tutor or a mentor. The following case study indicates a typical response to these questions.

Gaining access and ethical approval

Craig is a student nurse working in a hospital and studying a Project 2000 course. As part of the course he has to conduct a small research project. He wants to evaluate the effectiveness of the lifestyle advice given by nurses to patients who have suffered from a heart attack. He wants to find out specifically what type of advice nurses give, whether this is appropriate and how effective it is in influencing lifestyle choices.

Craig first approaches the ward sister of the coronary care ward to see if it would be acceptable to conduct his research on her ward. He takes with him a written summary of his research which includes the following points:

● an explanation of what he wants to do (as above)

- that he would like to design a health education package of lifestyle advice as a result of his findings

- that the effective elements of current advice given by nurses would be used as the basis of the package

- that the package would enhance the advice given to patients

- that a questionnaire (a copy of which he encloses) would be used to collect the data from both nurses and patients.

Once the sister has agreed to allow Craig to use her ward, he sends a copy of the summary, together with the questionnaires, to the senior manager of the hospital and asks permission for his research to be considered by the hospital ethics committee.

The senior manager sends Craig a form to be completed for ethical approval. Craig completes the form and returns it to the address given. One month later Craig receives a letter from the ethical committee stating that his proposal has been accepted on the condition that he amends three of the questions on the questionnaire.

Craig changes the questions as suggested, returns the revised questionnaire with the form to the ethics committee and two weeks later is given permission to proceed with his research.

This case study shows how important it is to allow plenty of time in which to gain permission. You need to ensure that you start early in trying to gain ethical approval. In Craig's case this took six weeks because he was required to revise his questionnaire. This is not unusual. Even if your proposal is straightforward, ethics committees may meet infrequently. You may have just missed a committee at the time you apply, which could delay your proposal by three weeks or more.

3: Selecting a target group

Once you have gained access to the organisation of your choice you then need to decide precisely who is going to be the target for your study. If the organisation is small and you want to use a survey approach, you may wish to use the whole study population of people within the organisation rather than a sample of them. This is called a 'population sample' and is really the only way of ensuring that your findings are representative of the whole study population. It may not be possible, however, to collect data from the entire population within the organisation. If you intend to use qualitative, in-depth interviews it would be preferable in any case to use a small number of respondents – probably less than ten.

If you do wish to use a sample that is *representative* of the population you will need to consider whether to use a probability or a non-probability sample.

Probability sampling: *A type of sampling strategy that assures each member of a population has an equal chance of being selected.*

A **probability sample** is so called because it ensures that each member of the population stands an equal chance of being included in the sample. All the variables naturally distributed throughout the population are distributed throughout the sample. This means that the sample is representative of the population of which it is a part, in respect of the variables under study. A probability sample (such as a simple or stratified random sample) is the strongest of these two categories of sampling and the one that you should be aiming to achieve.

ACTIVITY 29   ALLOW 5 MINUTES

We have just defined probability sampling. Write down what you think would be a definition of non-probability sampling.

Commentary

Non-probability sampling: *A type of sampling strategy in which there is no assurance that each member of the population has an equal chance of being selected.*

Non-probability sampling gives no assurance that every member of the population being studied stands an equal chance of being included in the sample. Naturally occurring variables within the population of which the sample is a part, may not be evenly distributed throughout the sample under study and, therefore, it may not be representative of the population. For example, a convenience sample of people who happen to be available and are willing to participate in the research may have certain characteristics which are different from the rest of the population. This introduces bias in the research findings and would reduce the credibility of your research findings.

Sub-categories of sampling strategies

Even though we have to accept that it is not always possible to achieve the best sample when researching human beings, within these two broad categories of probability and non-probability sampling there are sub-categories of sampling strategies. This means that within each of these categories you can still select the strongest sampling frame.

ACTIVITY 30   ALLOW 20 MINUTES

Look at the table below and, when you've read the descriptions, indicate whether you think it is a probability or a non-probability sample by the letters 'p' or 'np'.

Type of sample	Explanation and example
	Researcher allocates every individual a number from 1-200, then selects 50 numbers randomly for use as a sample. For example, a random sample of 50 new mothers might be selected from a population of 200 to administer the Edinburgh Post-natal Depression Scale (EPNDS).
	Researcher divides 200 people into identifiable groups (for example, different age groups, previous history of depression) then takes a systematic random sample from each group.
	Researcher can only access a small number of mothers, therefore only those attending a post-natal support group are used. Used for practical and logistical reasons.
	A health visitor distributes the EPNDS to those mothers on her caseload who are willing to participate.Participants are those who volunteer or who happen to be around.
	Researcher selects a sample that is a replica of total population, then asks the health visitor to select an appropriate sample.

Commentary

Your completed table should look like the one below. We have also filled in the names the subject categories of the sampling strategy described.

Type of sample	Explanation and example
Random p	Researcher allocates every individual a number from 1-200, then selects 50 numbers randomly for use as a sample. For example, a random sample of 50 new mothers might be selected from a population of 200 to administer the Edinburgh Post-natal Depression Scale (EPNDS).
Stratified p	Researcher divides 200 people into identifiable groups (for example, different age groups, previous history of depression) then takes a systematic random sample from each group.

Cluster	
p	Researcher can only access a small number of mothers, therefore only those attending a post-natal support group are used.Used for practical and logistical reasons.
Convenience	
n/p	A health visitor distributes the EPNDS to those mothers on her caseload who are willing to participate. Participants are those who volunteer or who happen to be around.
Quota	
n/p	Researcher selects a sample that is a replica of total population, then asks the health visitor to select an appropriate sample.

The information in the table above is hierarchical, with the sampling techniques at the top of the table being more powerful than the examples at the bottom. The ideal will always be a random sample because it's more representative of the population – providing, that is, that the sample is large enough to be representative. The size of the sample is always of great concern. As a general rule it is wise to use as large a sample as is possible within the constraints of the study. If you are dividing your subjects into experimental and control groups, you will need at least ten in each group. For survey research you would be wise to aim for 40 or more questionnaires. If you are forced to use a non-probability sample (for example, if your population is small or hard to reach) it is best to use a convenience sample and to make sure that you acknowledge the limitations of this in your research.

Strengths and weaknesses of the different sampling techniques

The strengths and weaknesses of the different sampling frames are listed in the table below.

Sampling frame	Strengths	Weaknesses
Probability	Suitable for both qualitative and quantitative methods Representative of the population of which the sample is a part	Can be difficult to obtain if population is small May be unrealistic if small sample size is required
Non-probability	Suitable for both qualitative and quantitative methods Can be used for small populations and small sample sizes Easier to acquire because large populations are not needed	Not representative of the population of which it is a part The results can't be relied upon

Quantitative methods require sampling techniques higher up the hierarchy such as surveys or experimental research. For experimental research you would need to use a random sample if at all possible and to randomly distribute the sample into two groups.

Qualitative researchers will find the techniques lower down the hierarchy sufficiently accurate. For example, if you wish to find out whether 'non-directive counselling' is a more effective treatment for post-natal depression than anti-depressants, you would need a random sample which you would then randomly assign to two groups – the 'anti-depressant' group and the 'non-directive counselling' group. Alternatively, if you wanted to determine the incidence of post-natal depression in a particular area you would gain the most reliable results by distributing, for example, the EPNDS to a random sample of the population. However, if you wanted to discover how people experience their depression – what coping strategies they employed and what family support was available –then in-depth interviews of a small convenience sample would be more reasonable.

Qualitative researchers can also use a **purposive sample**. This is discussed in Unit 1. This is a non-probability sample in which the sample is selected on the basis of a particular variable that the researcher is studying. For example, if you were interested in how new fathers experienced the transition to parenthood, you would need to interview a small sample of new fathers whom you would select because they were willing to be interviewed. This involves personal judgement on the part of the researcher about which respondents would be most representative of the population of which they are a part.

The following case study illustrates the use of the stratified random sample.

Stratified random sample

Jim is an occupational health nurse in a large hospital. He has noticed that during the past year there seems to be an increase in the number of nurses taking sick leave due to back injuries. He is aware that an in-service training programme on 'lifting' was implemented two years ago. He decides to conduct a research study to find out whether:

- the incidence of sick leave due to back pain has increased

- the number of nurses who have taken sick leave due to back pain actually attended the in-service training sessions

- those who did attend the sessions changed their lifting technique and in what ways.

The incidence of back pain is discovered by examining the statistics in the hospital records for the whole population of nurses in the hospital. The population of nurses is then stratified into all those who attended the sessions (including those on sick leave) and those who did not. Jim then takes a random sample of those who attended the sessions so that he can distribute a questionnaire asking them about any changes in their lifting technique.

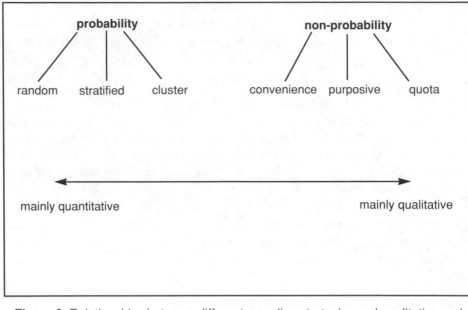

Figure 8: Relationships between different sampling strategies and qualitative and quantitative research

Figure 8 illustrates the relationships between the different sampling strategies and qualitative and quantitative research.

When you decide which sampling strategy to use in your own research project you need to select the most appropriate one – and this will be governed by the research method you choose. A qualitative methodology such as in-depth interviews allows you to use weaker sampling strategies such as a purposive sample.

Your approach to evaluation (for example, a goal-orientated, or user-orientated approach) will also influence your decision.

If you are using a decision-focused approach, the decision-makers may not be impressed by findings that are not representative of the population. You would need to use a probability sampling method, unless, of course, you are conducting a qualitative study.

The issue of representativeness also applies to the experimental approach and, to a certain extent, to the goal-orientated approach. For example, you will not be sure whether the goals of the programme have been achieved if your sample size is too small or your sampling strategy too weak.

If you are using either a user-orientated approach or a responsive approach you can be more flexible with your sampling because these approaches to evaluative research rely more heavily on qualitative methods.

If you want to state at the end of your research that changes need to be made in the area studied as a result of your findings, this will have little impact if your sample is inadequate for the type of research you have selected.

ALLOW 15 MINUTES

Indicate which sampling method is used in each of the following case studies.

Example	Type of sample
Andrew is a paediatric nurse and is evaluating the success of the use of nurses' own clothes rather than uniforms. He is particularly interested in the views of parents about whether they feel able to identify nurses easily and whether they feel that the new dress code breaks down professional barriers. He distributes a questionnaire to parents when they visit their children. He is unable to give a questionnaire to all parents because he is not always on duty when they visit. His sample is therefore limited to parents who are available when he is on duty.	
Julie is a midwife who wants to evaluate the effectiveness of an ante-natal class in which partners are actively encouraged to help the women with breathing exercises. Julie selects all the women who delivered with their partners present during the same month. She divides them into those whose partners attended the ante-natal class and those whose partners did not attend. She then distributes a questionnaire to a random sample of each group asking them about the effectiveness of the help and support given to them by their partners during labour.	
Fay is a social worker who is wanting to evaluate the success of a new programme to support single mothers in managing their household on a limited income and gaining access to scarce resources. She therefore interviews all the single mothers on her caseload who have used the service and are willing to be interviewed.	

John is a school nurse who is interested in the perceptions of young adolescents about healthy eating. He particularly wants to increase the knowledge level of adolescents about diet and therefore distributes questionnaires to one class of pupils in one of the schools he visits, at the beginning and end of a series of sessions devoted to healthy eating.

Commentary

Andrew used a convenience sample. Julie used a stratified random sample. Fay's sample was purposive. John used a cluster sample.

4: Deciding upon type of information and how to collect it

Once you have chosen your sampling method you are in a position to collect your data. Now you need to develop your actual instrument for data collection. The methods of data collection were discussed in Session Four of Unit 1 (Clifford, Carnwell and Harkin, 1996). Methods of collecting data for qualitative research were discussed in Unit 2 (Clifford, 1996).

Figure 9 shows the methods of data collection used within quantitative and qualitative approaches.

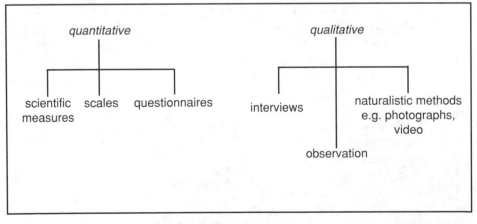

Figure 9: A contrast of the data collection methods used within quantitative and qualitative approaches to research

The most common data collection methods used for quantitative research are **questionnaires** and **scales**. Scientific measurements like blood pressure or temperature measurements may also be used. For the researcher interested in using observation methods in quantitative research, score sheets can be used to measure the number of occasions respondents engage in a particular type of behaviour. This approach could be used in the field of learning disabilities, for example measuring the number of occasions clients exhibit certain behaviours following certain interventions from staff. This would help to establish which interventions are most effective in minimising challenging behaviour.

The qualitative researcher is more likely to use **interviews** and **naturalistic observation** because these help the researcher to avoid influencing or contaminating the research by his or her presence. For the qualitative researcher data is 'free flowing' and undisturbed and the contents of the black box are out on display.

Before we discuss methods of data collection any further you will need to refresh your memory about questionnaires and interviews.

ACTIVITY 32　　ALLOW **15** MINUTES

Read the sections on Questionnaire design, Interviews and Observations in Session Four of Unit 1 (Clifford, Carnwell and Harkin, 1997) and the discussion of Interviews and Observation in Unit 2 (Clifford, 1997). Now write down in the table below the advantages and limitations of questionnaires, interviews and observations.

	Advantages	Limitations
Questionnaires		
Interviews		
Observations		

Commentary

Your answer to this activity should be similar to the table below.

	Advantages	Limitations
Questionnaires	Inexpensive Can gather a lot of data quickly and efficiently Easy to analyse Anonymity is likely to ensure honest response	Difficult to design Forced-response questions may not reflect what the respondent feels No opportunity to clarify ambiguous questions for respondent Return rate often low
Interviews	Can obtain information quickly Respondent can seek clarification of ambiguous questions Interviewer can clarify ambiguous responses	Respondents may say what they think interviewer wants to hear Accurate recording of data during interview Interviewer bias
Observations	Researcher can gain first-hand observation of situation	**Hawthorne effect** Observer bias

Hawthorne effect: *Also known as the 'experimenter effect' in which the subjects alter their behaviour because of their awareness of participating in the study.*

Questionnaires

If you decide to use questionnaires to collect your data you will need to decide what *type* of questionnaire to use. You could use an open-ended questionnaire, in which you ask a question and the respondents answer in their own words. Alternatively, you could develop a questionnaire comprising closed questions from which respondents select a given answer. A questionnaire combining both approaches could also be used.

ACTIVITY 33 ALLOW **15** MINUTES

Write down in the table below what you think the strengths and weaknesses of open and closed questions are.

	Advantages	Disadvantages
Open		
Closed		

Commentary

Advantages and disadvantages of open and closed questions are shown in the table below.

	Advantages	Disadvantages
Open	easy to construct	difficult to analyse
	richer and fuller	needs time from respondent
	freedom for respondent	requires written fluency
Closed	easy to analyse	difficult to construct
	efficient (respondent's time)	superficial
	no need to be articulate	bias – respondent forced to choose response which may not reflect their view

Once you have decided what type of questions you wish to ask you need to take care in actually formulating the questions. The checklist shown in *Figure 10* gives you an idea of points to consider when designing a questionnaire. The checklist applies to both open and closed-ended questionnaires.

Questionnaire checklist

1 Do you know what to do with the information you gain from each question?

2 Are you sure you need every one of the questions?

3 Does each question help you to answer your research question, hypothesis or problem?

4 Are your questions informed by current knowledge on the subject, for example, information gained from your review of the literature?

5 Are the questions short enough to avoid confusion?

6 Are there any 'double-barrelled' questions containing two distinct concepts? For example 'Do you like grapes or would you prefer apples?' could be altered to 'Indicate which of the following you prefer: apples/grapes'.

7 Have you used any technical terms that your respondents might not understand?

8 Have you used language that your respondents will understand – you need to write for the least educated respondents in your population.

---

9 Have you asked any leading questions that suggest a particular kind of answer? For example, 'Do you agree that all births should take place in hospital?' This could be replaced with 'Please indicate by ticking the appropriate box where you think babies should be born:

hospital □

home □

10 Have you avoided identifying an attitude with a prestigious person? For example, 'Princess Diana supports AIDS charities, how do you feel about them?'

11 Have you created a tone of tolerance towards questions that deal with socially unacceptable behaviour? For example, 'Many teenagers are acting irresponsibly by engaging in sexual activity. Do you think that parents should be blamed for this?' This could be replaced with ' What role do you think parents should play in encouraging teenagers to act responsibly in sexual relationships?'

Figure 10: Checklist of points to consider when designing questionnaires

Even the most competent researcher can produce questionnaires that are ambiguous. This is the reason why pilot tests are used. When you finally construct a questionnaire for your data collection do ensure that you pilot it on a group of people who resemble the respondents – about 10 people is normally sufficient. Piloting helps to ensure that the questionnaire has 'content validity' – that is, that it is successful in measuring what it is intended to measure.

Closed-ended questions

If you decide to use closed-ended questions in your questionnaire you can choose between a variety of types of question formats. We will only consider here the ones that are most useful to evaluative research. These are:

- dichotomous questions

- multiple choice questions

- rank-order questions.

Dichotomous questions are the simplest measurement and mean the choice between 'yes' and 'no'. They can be used throughout a questionnaire to discover whether or not respondents were satisfied with a specific element of a service. For example, you may ask the question: 'Were you satisfied with the care you received in hospital?'

Yes □   No □

Multiple choice questions give respondents a choice of answers. For example, if you were evaluating your services for children and their families on a paediatric ward you may ask parents: 'How important is it to you that nurses are specially trained in children's nursing in addition to their initial nurse training?'

The respondent can select from one of the following responses:

- extremely important

- very important

- fairly important

- not at all important.

Rank-order questions can be used when you would like respondents to rank responses in order of priority. For example, if you were evaluating the quality of life for people with learning disabilities in the community you might wish to find out which values are important to them from a range of responses. An example of this sort of question would be:

'Please indicate the order of importance of these values to you by placing 1 by the most important, 2 by the next most important and so on.

- contact with family

- having friends

- going shopping

- living in an ordinary house

- having my own bedroom.'

Measurement scales

An alternative to using closed-ended questions is to use one of a variety of different measurement scales.

Likert scales are the most common method of measuring attitudes. They consist of several statements to which respondents express their level of agreement or disagreement. An example of a Likert scale is a selection of statements like the following.

(**SA** means 'strongly agree', **A** means 'agree', **U** means 'unsure', **D** means 'disagree' and **SD** means 'strongly disagree'.)

		SA	A	U	D	SD
- 1	Abortions should be made illegal.	☐	☐	☐	☐	☐
+2	Professional counselling should be available for people who have abortions.	☐	☐	☐	☐	☐
+3	Nurses should not be allowed to refuse to nurse someone who has had an abortion.	☐	☐	☐	☐	☐
- 4	People who have abortions deserve what they get.	☐	☐	☐	☐	☐

The + and – signs at the beginning of each statement refer to the positive or negative nature of the statement. Equal numbers of positive and negative statements are used. Their order is mixed up to prevent bias arising from respondents just placing ticks under one particular column, rather than thinking carefully about their response and using more than one column.

When designing Likert scales you should remember always to use *statements* not questions. If you need a question mark at the end of your sentence then it is inappropriate for a Likert scale. For example, 'Do you think that people who refuse to treat AIDS patients are irresponsible?' would be replaced with 'People who refuse to treat AIDS patients are irresponsible'. The first of these sentences is a question, whereas the second is a statement.

You should also ensure that positively and negatively worded statements are randomly distributed within the scale. Never present a list of negative statements followed by a list of positive statements. Mixing them up reduces bias in your results.

Before you can analyse the results of a scale you need to ensure that it does in fact measure **attitudes**. A common failing is for students to mistake **attitudes** for **knowledge**. It is not the purpose of a Likert scale to test knowledge. Knowledge is something that you either know or don't know. It is not something about which you can indicate agreement.

Take the following statement as an example. 'HIV is transmitted through body fluids.' This is a fact. You could use this statement to test whether someone had this knowledge, but you would need to use a dichotomous scale of 'true/false' here rather than a Likert scale.

ACTIVITY 34

ALLOW **10** MINUTES

Identify the positively worded and negatively worded statements in the Likert scale below. Write a + or - before each statement to indicate your answer.

	SA	A	U	D	SD
1 Nurses should be able to refuse to care for people with AIDS if they wish.	☐	☐	☐	☐	☐
2 People with AIDS should be nursed with the same compassion as any other patient.	☐	☐	☐	☐	☐
3 People who are HIV positive should have the same rights to a mortgage as other people.	☐	☐	☐	☐	☐
4 People with AIDS deserve what they get.	☐	☐	☐	☐	☐
5 People who contract HIV through blood transfusions should have special services.	☐	☐	☐	☐	☐
6 Health professionals who are HIV positive should be allowed to continue working providing appropriate precautions are taken.	☐	☐	☐	☐	☐

	SA	A	U	D	SD
7 Nurses should always wear special protective clothing when in contact with AIDS patients.	☐	☐	☐	☐	☐
8 Specialised bereavement counselling should be offered to partners of people who have died of AIDS.	☐	☐	☐	☐	☐

Commentary

The positive statements are 2, 3, 6 and 8. The negative statements are 1, 4, 5 and 7.

ACTIVITY 35   ALLOW 30 MINUTES

Design a 10 item Likert scale relevant to your area of practice. When you have designed your scale ask about ten of your colleagues to complete it.

Commentary

It would be a good idea to discuss the responses to your questionnaire with your tutor and mentor as well as other students. In particular, it would be useful to discuss any statements that seem to be ambiguous and possible changes you could make to them.

ACTIVITY 36   ALLOW 20 MINUTES

When you have successfully piloted your scale on your colleagues you will need to know how to make sense of their responses.

People who agree with positively worded statements should get higher total scores than those who disagree.

1 Start by scoring the positive statements from 1-5, with 5 given to those who strongly agree and working backwards until you give 1 to those who strongly disagree.

2 Reverse the scoring for the negative statements, with 1 given to those who strongly agree and 5 to those who strongly disagree.

3 Total the scores for each respondent and write the total score for each respondent at the bottom of the questionnaire.

Commentary

The questionnaire should be designed in such a way that respondents who gain high scores have a more positive attitude than those who gain low scores. You may find that some items are endorsed equally by those with high total scores and those with low total scores. For example, both the respondents with positive and negative attitudes may consistently indicate uncertainty with a certain statement. This means that these items are either irrelevant to the attitude being measured or ambiguously worded. You should therefore exclude them from the final version of the questionnaire.

In the Likert scale in *Figure 11*, √ and × refer to two respondents who have completed a Likert scale. You will notice that the respondent with the most positive attitude (√) gains a higher score throughout most of the scale. They gain a total score of 35 in comparison to ×'s score of 14.

Two statements (1 and 5) are endorsed equally by both respondents. This may, of course, be a coincidence. However, if this occurred with a larger sample of respondents we would have to conclude that these two questions were ambiguous because they do not measure what they are supposed to measure. Statement 1, for example, could be regarded as an ethical issue, with which agreement does not necessarily reflect a negative attitude. Equally, respondents agreeing with statement 5 may not wish to discriminate between groups of AIDS patients, but may recognise the different needs of certain groups.

	SA	A	U	D	SD	√	×
-1 Nurses should be able to refuse to care for people with AIDS if they wish.			×√			3	3
+2 People with AIDS should be nursed with the same compassion as any other patient.	√			×		5	2
+3 People who are HIV positive should have the same rights to a mortgage as other people.	√				×	5	1
-4 People with AIDS deserve what they get.	×				√	5	1
-5 People who contract HIV through blood transfusions should have special services.			×√			3	3
+6 Health professionals who are HIV positive should be allowed to continue working providing appropriate precautions are taken.		√			×	4	1
-7 Nurses should wear special protective clothing when nursing AIDS patients.	×				√	5	1
+8 Specialised bereavement counselling should be offered to partners of people who have died of AIDS.	√		×			5	2
	TOTAL√ = 35 × = 14						

Figure 11: A Likert scale showing the scores of two respondents – × and √

Likert scales are commonly used to measure a change in attitude following some educational input. If you used this method you would need to test the respondents both before and after the intervention.

An example of a situation in which a Likert scale could be used in evaluative research would be to evaluate the satisfaction of users with a new service. A list of statements indicating the attributes service providers think they are providing could be designed and respondents could be asked to state their strength of agreement regarding whether these attributes were actually present and whether they were satisfied with them.

The semantic differential scale is of great value in evaluative research. It too measures respondents' strength of feeling, this time along a continuum. Respondents are asked to place a tick or cross in an appropriate place on a linear scale. For example:

'How would you rate the session on Looking After Your Heart?'

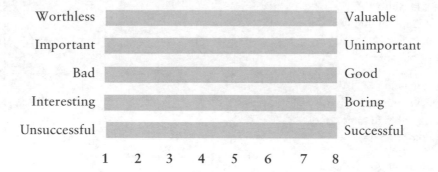

Worthless		Valuable
Important		Unimportant
Bad		Good
Interesting		Boring
Unsuccessful		Successful

1 2 3 4 5 6 7 8

When designing a semantic differential scale you need to ensure that adjectives are appropriate for the concepts being used and for the information sought. Information from your review of the literature should enable you to determine suitable adjectives. As in the Likert scale, the direction of the adjective pairs is randomly reversed to prevent bias and the positively worded adjective is normally associated with the higher score. Scores for each respondent are totalled to find out how valuable the session was.

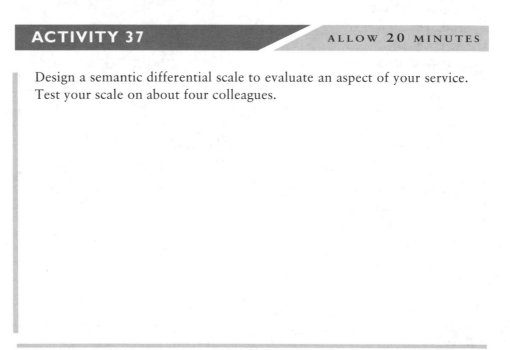

ACTIVITY 37

ALLOW 20 MINUTES

Design a semantic differential scale to evaluate an aspect of your service. Test your scale on about four colleagues.

Commentary

How successful were you in designing your scales? Did your respondents understand what was required? Were there any ambiguities in the design of your statements or adjectives? It would be useful to compare your scales with those produced by other students as the variety of adjectives that can be used is surprising. Discussing your scale with a tutor will also be useful to ensure that you have understood properly what is required of you.

You should by now be able to design a questionnaire or scale for use in collecting data. You may, however, decide that this is an inappropriate means for collecting your data and think interviewing would be a more successful method for your study. It is to this that we now turn.

Interviewing

The interview method was discussed extensively in Unit 2, Session Three (Clifford, 1997). Before we consider interviewing in relation to evaluative research it would be useful for you to review this discussion.

ACTIVITY 38
ALLOW 1 HOUR

Read the sections entitled 'Types of interview', 'Using interviews in research', 'Doing interviews' and the section on 'Focus group interviews' in Clifford (1997).

Make brief notes under the following headings of points you need to remember when using the interview method.

1   Types of interviews.

2   Planning and conducting interviews.

3   Closing the interview.

4   Using focus group interviews.

Commentary

1 You probably identified the following types of interview:

- structured interviews
- semi-structured interviews
- low-structured interviews.

2 When carrying out interviews you need to plan in advance:

- the type of interview you intend to use
- how you intend to record what has been said, for example making notes or using a tape-recorder
- how to gain a rapport with respondents
- what to tell respondents about your research
- where you will carry out the interview.

3 When you close the interview you will need to make any arrangements necessary to follow up with respondents or to verify that your interpretation is a faithful account of their true feelings. You will also need to decide whether or not to send respondents a copy of the final research findings.

4 Focus group interviews, which involve a group of about 8-12 respondents, focus on the views of the group as a whole. If you use this method you will need to be careful in documenting the interview. A lot of information is likely to be forthcoming in a short amount of time and you could have difficulty sorting out who said what. A tape-recorder may prove useful. You will also need to be aware of whether the views of some members of the group are not represented because other members dominate the group.

It is always useful to devise a schedule before you start interviewing, and in most cases – as with questionnaires – the content of your schedule should be influenced by your review of the literature.

Structured interview schedules

Structured interview schedules are similar to questionnaires in that they provide a standardised set of items with predetermined wording of both questions and alternative responses. When you use this type of interview you need to ensure that all subjects respond to the same questions in the same order and have the same set of options for their responses. This standardisation helps to reduce 'interviewer bias' – where respondents may be influenced by the way the interviewer phrases questions to give responses that they think will please the interviewer. Possible interviewer bias is one of the weaknesses of the interview method.

Semi-structured interviews

In semi-structured interviews you are able to follow up some of the leads presented by the respondent whilst also following your schedule. This can be particularly pertinent when evaluating your service provision. For example, a question in the structured schedule may ask 'how satisfied are you with the timing of the visits from your social worker?' If the respondent answers 'totally dissatisfied' you may wish to enquire further to find out more about this dissatisfaction. A semi-structured interview could simply consist of a list of topics to be covered, specifying only the order in which they should be covered.

Although this method allows more flexibility for the researcher, it can introduce researcher bias, both in the framing of questions and in the interpretation of data. Because the data will be so diverse the researcher will need to interpret the meaning of the responses and this interpretation could introduce bias into the research.

Low-structured interviews

This type of interview may be the preferred method if you wish to discover respondents' perceptions of the world without imposing your own view by posing predetermined questions. The method uses a conversational style and is suitable for naturalistic settings. For example, you might wish to observe nurses during a range of shifts to see whether the interaction with patients varies across shifts. You might also want to talk to nurses about how they feel at various points in their shift. You would be able to converse with them in a natural way (within the context of their normal working day) so that you would be more likely to capture their real feelings rather than feelings they might have 'rehearsed'. Low-structured interviews are therefore particularly suited to a user-orientated or responsive approach.

Focus group interviews

In evaluating your services you may wish to gain the views of several individuals in a short amount of time. You might have a limited time period to collect data and feel that your potential respondents would respond well in a group interview. For example, women in a hostel for battered women might feel more relaxed in a group situation if you are asking questions about services provided for them. In focus group interviews, the interviewer uses an interview schedule to lead the discussion and then records the responses as they occur.

Using interviews for critical research

Low-structured interviews and focus group interviews are well suited to critical research methods in which the researcher becomes closely involved with participants. Dialogue is important in this type of research because it is the means through which the reality of the participants' experience is uncovered. Guba and Lincoln (1994) suggest that this dialogue should be 'dialectical' in nature. The researcher and respondent enter into a two-way dialogue designed to ensure that the researcher gains an accurate account of the lived experience of the respondent uncontaminated by the researcher's own experiences and prejudices.

If you decide to use this method, you will constantly **interrogate** the respondent as to whether you have understood correctly what has been said or implied in their statements, rather than simply asking questions for which a straightforward answer is required. This constant checking of understanding ensures that you are not acting on your own assumptions or prior experience.

Interrogation: A statement in question form which seeks to identify a gap in knowledge.

ACTIVITY 39   ALLOW **10** MINUTES

Write down two examples of research situations where the researcher's own gender or ethnic background might make him or her introduce bias into the data.

Commentary

Our responses to any situation are obviously conditioned by our life and work experiences. Two examples of situations where bias might arise follow.

- A female researcher who had spent a lot of time interviewing battered women and who identified with her interviewees might find it hard to be objective if called upon to research battered men.

- A researcher brought up in Britain might find it hard to lay aside his or her own feelings when interviewing women from other cultural backgrounds who had experienced female circumcision.

Interviews are not always easy to administer because you can't anticipate how interviewees will respond to you. Professional researchers are trained in interview techniques and become skilled in putting respondents at ease and in using good communication skills. Since you won't have the benefit of this training you will need to prepare your interview schedule carefully and to practise your interview skills on a colleague or relative before collecting data from users. You should also remember the ethical considerations involved when dealing with sensitive information and reassure respondents that you will not disclose anything that is said to you during the interview.

The points in the checklist in *Figure 12* should be borne in mind when undertaking interviews.

Interviewing checklist

1 When using a *structured* interview schedule:

- follow the wording of the question precisely

- repeat the question if required, but do not rephrase or explain the meaning of the question

- don't read from the schedule – this may make the respondent feel uncomfortable or give the impression that you lack confidence

- if a list of alternative responses is required show the list to the respondent to give them time to think of a response.

2 In *structured* or *semi-structured* interviews record responses to open-ended questions in full without paraphrasing.

3 In *semi-structured* interviews probe to elicit more information. For example, 'Go on', 'How do you mean?', 'Is there anything else?'.

Figure 12: Interviewing checklist.

ACTIVITY 40　　　　ALLOW 15 MINUTES

1 Decide which of the types of interview discussed in this session would be most appropriate to your proposed research and develop an interview schedule suitable for this purpose.

2 Use your interview schedule to interview at least one of your colleagues. (Your schedule will probably be designed for service users but you won't be able to use it on them without gaining ethical approval. Testing your schedule on colleagues will allow you to check how well you conduct an interview and that the questions you ask are appropriate.)

3 After you have completed the interview ask your colleague to give you some feedback on your interview technique, using the points from the interview checklist above according to which kind of interview you used.

4 List in the space below:

- the things you did well in the interview (as stated by your colleague)

- the things you could improve upon.

Commentary

How successful were you in your interviewing? If you think you need to improve your skills try discussing any problems you have with a tutor and have another go at conducting an interview later on.

Observation methods

You may find that observation methods would be more appropriate to your research than either questionnaires or interviews. For example, you might wish to observe people in a naturalistic setting as part of a responsive approach to evaluation, or, if you are using a goal-orientated approach for your evaluative research, you might need to observe specific changes in behaviour to determine whether or not a programme had achieved its goals.

'Observation research' is the systematic selection, observation and recording of behaviours and settings relevant to the research problem.

ACTIVITY 41

Return to the discussion of observation research in Session Three of Clifford (1997) and make brief notes under the following headings.

1 Structured observation.

2 Semi-structured observation.

3 Unstructured observation.

4 Ethical issues in observation research.

Commentary

1 Structured observation requires that the researcher specify the types of observations which will be recorded *before* the observation actually takes place. If you decide to use this method you will probably decide on the specific characteristics or categories of behaviour you are interested in during the planning stage of your study.

Structured observation

Louise is a health visitor who has recently set up a market stall in a local indoor market to distribute health advice and health education leaflets to the local population. Because the highest cause of death in the area is coronary heart disease in middle-aged men, Louise hopes that men in mid-life will pick up some of her leaflets on prevention of heart disease, and take advantage of the blood pressure test she is offering. In addition, because the incidence of breast cancer in women is increasing in the area, Louise offers advice and leaflets about self-examination of the breast for women. Although these two subjects form her two large poster displays, Louise also offers health advice on a range of other matters.

Because Louise has only just set up her stall she can't really ask her clients to complete a questionnaire regarding the value of the service provided. This would not be appropriate anyway because each client probably only spends a few minutes at the stall. During the early stages, therefore, she carries out evaluation using the observation method. Louise does a simple tally of all the people who approach her for information. For each person she records gender and approximate age. In addition, Louise categorises all the leaflets on display, (for example, diet, stress, sexual health, women's health, men's health) and then records the number of people from each age group and gender who pick up the different categories of leaflet.

This information, which is collected purely by structured observation, will enable Louise to assess how successful she has been in targeting different age groups and genders. Louise can then use this information to tailor her services to local needs and interests. If she is unsuccessful in targeting groups particularly in need of advice she can consider other ways of attracting their interest.

2　Semi-structured observation can be used when you don't need to be so prescriptive with your parameters of observation. Louise could have evaluated the effectiveness of the stall by observing the interest shown by different people in relation to health issues. Louise could define the variable of 'interest' using her own observation skills and professional judgement (such as asking questions, reading leaflets, discussing leaflets with a friend) rather than using pre-specified categories. This could be a more reliable method than counting the different groups who pick up different leaflets. Some people may collect a leaflet even though they are not really interested in it and may never read it. As the observation becomes less structured it also becomes more difficult to record and interpret.

3　Unstructured observation requires an even more intricate account of events than the semi-structured method. Louise would certainly need help in managing the stall if she chose to use this approach. She could then devote the entire time to writing down events as they occurred. The following box shows what Louise might have recorded during 30 minutes of observation.

Unstructured observation

10.00 am. A man in his 50s approaches the stall. He looks hesitant and seems to be encouraged as the health visitor smiles at him and points to some of the leaflets. He looks about two stone overweight and has a ruddy complexion. The health visitor asks him if he's interested in any health leaflets and advice. He says he's interested in heart disease because he had a minor heart attack a few months ago. The health visitor asks him if he would like his blood pressure taken. A rapport seems to develop as he readily agrees. He says his blood pressure was quite high a month ago and that he is taking tablets to lower it. The health visitor tells him that it is still slightly high and that a visit to his own doctor would be a good idea. She asks if he was given advice about lifestyle following his heart attack. He says he was advised to cut down on fats, sugar and carbohydrate and to stop smoking. He says his diet is much healthier but that he has only managed to reduce his cigarettes from 30 to 10 per day because he has a stressful job. The health visitor asks if he has attended any stress management courses or other alternatives such as yoga or relaxation. He says he is not aware of any but would be willing to try. She gives him the telephone number of local groups and also suggests that afterwards he may benefit from attending a smoking cessation group run at the local health centre.

10.10 am. A woman in her 40s approaches and has obviously overheard the end of the conversation with the man in his 50s. She appears fit and confident. She mentions that she overheard the conversation about the smoking cessation group and says that it was the way that she managed to give up smoking a few months ago. She strongly recommends it to the man. The man then thanks the health visitor for the advice and departs.

10.15 am. A woman in her 20s starts flicking through the leaflets with vague interest. She seems particularly interested in a leaflet on cervical smears and sits down to read the leaflet. The woman in her 40s talks to the health visitor about breast cancer. She says that her sister died of breast cancer five years ago and that she is concerned about the increased risk to herself. The health visitor gives her a leaflet on self-examination of the breast and explains the leaflet to her. She advises her to seek an appointment with the practice nurse if she would like a practical demonstration of the technique.

10.25 am. The woman reading the leaflets on cervical smears catches the eye of the health visitor, but abruptly looks away as though she is trying to avoid direct contact. She continues reading the leaflet and then picks up a leaflet on sexual health.

> 10.30 am. As the woman concludes the discussion on breast examination, the health visitor tidies up the leaflets on sexual health and appears to be making herself available to the woman reading the leaflets. The woman seems not to be interested in any discussion – she takes the leaflets and leaves.

4   Ethical issues are particularly important in observation research because people being observed may feel uncomfortable in the researcher's presence. In the box above, the last person to look at the leaflets seemed to want to avoid conversation with the health visitor. We cannot be sure whether this was because of the nature of the subject, the presence of the researcher or some other reason. Whatever the reason, the woman could have been deprived of some important health information and so it could be helpful for Louise to approach her to ask her if she could help her in any way.

Before you embark on using observation techniques you should decide how structured your observations need to be and how to overcome any ethical issues involved.

You may have recognised by now the strengths and weaknesses of the different types of observation. These are shown in the table below.

	Unstructured observation	Structured observation
Strengths	Provides a deep and rich understanding of human behaviour Allows the researcher to 'get inside' a situation.	Unawareness of the observer by participants and use of a structured category system improve control over research and reduce bias. Lack of emotional involvement of researcher enhances objectivity and therefore reduces bias. Use of checklists and other memory aids ensures accuracy of data and reduces memory distortions.
Weaknesses	Observer could influence behaviour and therefore bias the results. Inappropriate sampling of events or time periods (for example, during the night) when it is known that the behaviour or interest does not occur.	Understanding of human behaviour superficial and limited by categories defined by researchers. Requires careful planning of precise data to be collected and categories for observation.

	Unstructured observation	Structured observation
	Emotional involvement on the part of the observer may bias the results.	Requires a skilled observer to categorise behaviour as it occurs.
	Inaccuracy due to memory distortions.	

The next activity will help you to apply our discussion of observation methods to your practice.

ACTIVITY 42

ALLOW 20 MINUTES

1 Write down an area of your work that could be evaluated using observation methods.

2 State whether you would use a structured, semi-structured or unstructured approach and give reasons for your choice.

3 If you chose a structured or semi-structured approach state what categories of behaviour you would use – for example, type and speed of movement, non-verbal communication or signs of pain. Think about how precise your observations would need to be.

4 If you chose to use an unstructured approach state what type of events you are interested in and why.

5   Devise a sheet on which to record your observations.

Commentary

It would be useful for you to discuss your responses to this activity with other students or, if this is not possible, with a colleague or mentor.

1,2 and 3. An example of an area in which observation research could be used is in a child assessment unit. A new programme of 'gentle teaching' has been adopted and the researcher wishes to evaluate its effectiveness. The phenomena to be observed could fall into the following categories:

- non-verbal communication behaviours (expression, gesture, touch)

- activities, (eating habits, grooming)

- skill attainment and performance (skill in carrying out a learned task).

This observation would probably be very structured, with precise categories of behaviour, because the researcher is looking for very small improvements in specific behaviours (such as a reduction in hand flapping).

The researcher will probably be concealed behind a one-way mirror to prevent any bias arising from the awareness of the researcher's presence by the participants. You will need to decide in your own evaluation study whether it will be necessary to have a good deal of interaction with participants, as in participant observation, or whether you need to be discreet.

Your decision regarding structured or unstructured observations needs careful consideration *before* you start collecting your data. As well as deciding which structure to use in your observations, you also need to decide what type of sampling frame and what method you are going to use to *record* the data. You will need to consider the amount of time you can realistically spend observing. For example, would it be realistic to observe behaviour for the period of an entire shift? This could, of course, be essential if your research were concerned with types of behaviour and activities that vary at different points in a shift. However, this would generate a vast amount of data.

The recording of the behaviour is also important. You may have decided to use a naturalistic approach or you may have already defined your categories. The naturalistic approach might necessitate using a blank piece of paper for your 'field notes'. If you have decided to use a structured checklist you will also need a tally on which to record the *frequency* and *duration* of the behaviours. An example of a typical checklist and tally is shown in the table below.

Behaviour recorded for two-hour period 6-8 pm.

Behaviour	Frequency	Duration
Head banging	√√√	3 mins, 5 mins, 2 mins
Hand flapping	√√	10 mins, 2 mins
Self-destructive behaviour	√√	2 mins, 3 mins
Verbal abuse	√	5 mins

An alternative method of recording data is to use a video recorder. This would be appropriate for both structured or unstructured observations because it captures complex behaviour that could be missed by the observer. If you are carrying out naturalistic observation you can use videos to enhance your field notes. If you have used checklists, videos can help you to check the accuracy of coding, particularly if several different people have carried out the coding and have interpreted behaviours differently from each other.

Using records as data

So far we have discussed methods of data collection that require you to gain information from people. However, other types of data can be equally valuable. Suppose, for example, that you wanted to evaluate the effectiveness of a new triage system (a system of allocating patients to treatment categories according to the severity of their condition) to be introduced in an accident and emergency department (A&E). You could ask patients what they think about the system, but their perceptions might be distorted by many factors other than the effectiveness of triage (such as anxiety about informing a relative of their whereabouts, or about missing an appointment they have elsewhere). Another way you could measure the effectiveness of triage is through patient records. You could ask the A&E staff to record the following information both before and after the introduction of the triage system:

- the time of arrival of each patient

- the time of treatment or X-ray of each patient

- the diagnosis of each patient

- the category into which each patient had been allocated.

You could then compare the length of time between arrival and treatment for patients with different conditions before and after the introduction of the triage system. If triage was successful you would expect to find that:

- patients allocated to the 'severe' category are treated promptly

- patients allocated to the least severe category are treated less promptly

- patients with certain conditions are reliably allocated to certain categories.

This method gives you valuable data without having to worry about response bias or interview bias.

As we have seen, your research approach must use a method of data collection which is conducive to that approach. (See *Figure 13*.)

Evaluation approach	Data collection method
Experimental	Tests, scientific measurements, quantitative scales
Goal-orientated	Questionnaires, structured interviews, tests of performance such as knowledge gained following a health education programme, structured observations
Decision-focused	Questionnaires, interviews, documents, records, other methods determined by decision-maker
User-orientated	Interviews, naturalistic observation, open-ended questionnaires
Responsive	Interviews, naturalistic observation.

Figure 13: Data collection methods used within different evaluation approaches.

When you evaluate services there is a variety of sources of information (including observation, questionnaires, interviews and records) which can help to indicate the value of the service you provide. Your task as a researcher is to select the methods which will give you the most valuable information. Bear in mind that the approach you are using will influence your choice of methods for collecting data and never be afraid to use more than one method. For example, the use of hospital records would give you an objective account of the timing of treatments for different categories of patient. Since the main purpose of a triage system is to ensure that patients with more serious conditions are treated promptly, the use of records would certainly be valuable. However, a more accurate assessment of the effectiveness of triage might involve you in combining the use of records with interviewing patients to see how satisfied different categories of them were with the treatment they received.

By now you should have some insight into collecting data for your evaluation study. We will now consider how to go about analysing it once you have gathered it.

5: Analysing your data

In this unit we have discussed the two main types of research – qualitative and quantitative. Naturally, these two types of research generate two corresponding types of data:

- qualitative data
- quantitative data.

When you analyse your data from your evaluation study there will be three options open to you, depending on the type of research methods you have used. We will deal with each of these in turn.

Analysing qualitative data

You will find Unit 2, Session Four (Clifford, 1996) particularly useful in explaining how to analyse qualitative data. The following activity will assist you in revising your understanding of this subject.

Referring to Unit 2, Session Four (Clifford, 1996), write brief notes under the following headings.

1 Data display.

2 Data reduction.

3 Data interpretation.

Commentary

1 Data display involves transcribing in full all the data from interviews or observations so that they can be seen in their entirety. Since this is a very laborious process one soon learns not to collect too much data by avoiding lengthy interviews and observations, and large sample sizes.

2 Dealing with the data once they have been displayed is known as data reduction because it involves reducing the total amount into smaller, more manageable units in order to see patterns in the data more easily (Miles and Huberman, 1994). For example, although you are unlikely to see any patterns by glancing at an A4 page of typescript, once this has been broken down into manageable units you will be able to see trends much more quickly.

Sifting and sorting through a script in order to identify patterns is called content analysis. This process starts with collation of responses to a single question. Most data in qualitative research are complex because one respondent might cover several issues in a single answer to an open-ended question. When faced with this situation the researcher would need to break each sentence down into a smaller unit without losing the sense of what has been said and underline the key words in each sentence.

3   Once key words have been identified, data interpretation can begin. All the words with a common link are grouped by listing them or by drawing a concept map. It is important to remember that data interpretation is the researcher's *interpretation* of what the respondent has said. Categories will be devised from words used by respondents in order to interpret the data.

If you feel uncertain about any of the above commentary you should review the activities associated with Unit 2, Session Four again.

Observation data

Observation data can be quantitative or qualitative depending on whether the observations are divided into small units that are categorised numerically or large (naturalistic) observations of naturally occurring events that are recorded as field notes. If your observation data is naturalistic, your field notes will probably resemble an interview transcript when they are written in a prose format. This means that naturalistic data can be subjected to the same type of analysis as interview data. For example, imagine that you want to evaluate the effectiveness of skill mix in a child surveillance clinic. You observe nursery nurses' interactions with children and parents during a two-hour clinic and record your observations using field notes. In your analysis you may have particular themes that are relevant to your research question, such as the number of times nursery nurses engage in activities for which they are not qualified. Other data may be more 'free flowing' and you may wait until you read your notes before imposing themes on your data. You would therefore read your notes as you would an interview transcript and look for events that could be categorised and linked together by common themes. For example, you may notice that nursery nurses used similar ways of gaining the co-operation of children, which could be classified as 'rapport with children'. You may find also that the nursery nurses were very adept at disciplining children. Discipline could be classed under 'rapport with children' as it can be used as a means of gaining children's co-operation.

Since observation research is usually qualitative, statistics are not normally associated with it. However, if you were using a stopwatch to record your observations of the speed with which nurses of different levels of experience carried out different tasks you would end up with numerical scores, even though you had used an observation method. You could also record the number of times you observed nurses use touch to comfort patients, or how many times they used eye contact with patients. If your observations are divided into small categories which can be recorded numerically then descriptive statistics would be used to analyse the data. It might be interesting, however, to see whether nurses of higher grades use touch and eye contact more frequently than nurses of lower grades. We could *hypothesise* that there would be a *significant* difference between the different grades of nurses and could therefore subject our observation data to *inferential* statistics. We turn to the use of descriptive and inferential statistics next.

Analysing quantitative data

As you will probably recall, quantitative data is always subjected to some type of calculation, using either one or both of the two different types of statistic:

- descriptive statistics which *describe* the trends in the data, such as '50 per cent of respondents strongly agreed' and 'the mean score was 12'

- inferential statistics which enable us to draw conclusions from a set of data which can then be applied to a similar situation.

We will now briefly discuss each of these in turn as they apply to evaluative research. However, if you are unfamiliar with any of the content of this section you are advised to re-read Clifford et al (1997).

Descriptive statistics

Descriptive statistics are so-called because they *describe* the data. For example, 80 per cent of respondents may agree with a new system of care and 20 per cent may disagree. Descriptive statistics are normally presented in the form of tables, graphs, histograms and pie diagrams.

Researchers using descriptive statistics often refer to different types of average, namely the mean, median and mode. For example, the researcher might state that the mean average score among a group of respondents was 50. The mean average provides more information about the data than the other two and is therefore more powerful or accurate. It is necessary to distinguish between these three types of average because different statistical tests require the use of different types of average. For example, more powerful **parametric tests** normally require the use of the mean rather than the median or mode, whereas non-parametric tests allow the researcher to use the median or mode although the results will be less reliable.

Researchers also refer to the range and the standard deviation (SD). The range differentiates between the highest and lowest numbers in a set of figures. The standard deviation refers to the average degree of deviation of a set of scores from the mean. For example, an SD of 1.2 means that there is less deviation from the mean than an SD of 3.6. One would expect therefore that the scores with the SD of 1.2 are more clustered together than those with the SD of 3.6.

Parametric test: *A test to establish the parameters of a population usually based on the mean of the sample*

Inferential statistics

We need inferential statistics to help us to find out whether our findings are simply a matter of chance or whether there is a probability of them being correct. Inferential statistics rely on a hypothesis being formulated which the statistics will either support or reject.

A hypothesis is a statement of the predicted relationship between two or more variables. For example, 'pre-school children will develop a larger vocabulary if they attend a play group' states a relationship between the development of vocabulary (the dependent variable) which is dependent upon attendance at a play group (the independent variable). The hypothesis can be tested by comparing the number of words used by children who attend play group with the number used by those who do not. The two sets of scores (number of words) would then be subjected to a statistical test to see if there was a significant difference between them.

As in the above example, two variables are always stated in a hypothesis. These are:

- the independent variable which can be manipulated by the researcher (for example, a drug)

- the dependent variable which is dependent upon the independent variable (for example, a reduction in pain).

Every hypothesis should also be accompanied by a null hypothesis which contradicts (but is not the opposite of) the hypothesis. Whereas the hypothesis states that there is a relationship between the variables, the null hypothesis always refutes this claim, stating that there is no relationship between the variables, for example, 'there is no relationship between attendance at a play group and the development of vocabulary in the pre-school child'.

Before calculating data using inferential statistics it is necessary to select a significance level. This is often referred to as a 'p value' which refers to the probability of the findings being wrong (due to random error). A 'p' value of 0.05 (5 per cent) is normally considered acceptable.

It is also important to state the number of tails on the hypothesis before you analyse your results because this will affect the statistical test used. A one-tailed hypothesis always states one outcome in a hypothesis, e.g. that 'there will be an *improvement*...', 'recovery will be *faster* ...'. A two-tailed hypothesis gives two possible outcomes by merely stating that 'there will be a *difference* in...' – and the difference could be better or worse.

Tail: *The number of outcomes identified within a hypothesis – either one or two.*

You may recall from your reading of Unit 2 (Clifford 1997), that the type of statistical test you use is also determined by the level of data that you have collected. The table below shows the names given to the types of data collected.

Nominal	Yes/no male/female
Ordinal	Strongly agree to strongly disagree (Likert scale)
Interval/ratio	A percentage score

You should, by now, be familiar with some of the basic data-analysis procedures. Because it is important to decide how you intend to analyse your data when you first design your study, we now ask you to consider the types of data analysis you would use for the different evaluation approaches.

ACTIVITY 44 ALLOW 15 MINUTES

Look back at *Figure 13* illustrating the types of data collection used for different evaluation approaches.

The two lists shown below give the various evaluation approaches and methods of data analysis. Draw a connecting line between the relevant evaluation approaches and the relevant methods of data analysis. (The information in *Figure 13* will help you work these out.

Evaluation approach	Data analysis
Experimental	Mainly descriptive statistics of questionnaire data, possibly some inferential statistics if descriptive statistics reveal possible relationships between variables. Qualitative analysis used if decision-makers dictate the use of qualitative methods
Goal-orientated	Mainly qualitative analysis for interviews and observation Some descriptive statistics for questionnaires

Evaluation approach	Data analysis
Decision-focused	Descriptive and inferential statistics
User-orientated	Qualitative analysis
Responsive	Descriptive statistics, inferential statistics, possibly some qualitative analysis of interview data

Commentary

Your answer should match that shown in the table below, which is an extended version of *Figure 13*.

Completed table showing evaluation approaches, methods and analysis

Evaluation approach	Data collection method	Data analysis
Experimental	Tests, scientific measurements, quantitative scales	Descriptive and inferential statistics
Goal-orientated	Questionnaires, structured interviews, tests of performance such as knowledge gained following a health education programme, structured observations	Descriptive statistics, inferential statistics, possibly some qualitative analysis of interview data
Decision-focused	Questionnaires, interviews, documents, records, other methods determined by decision-makers	Mainly descriptive statistics of questionnaire data, possibly some inferential statistics if descriptive statistics reveal possible relationships between variables. Qualitative analysis used if decision-makers dictate the use of qualitative methods
User-orientated	Interviews, naturalistic observation, open-ended questionnaires	Mainly qualitative analysis for interviews and observation. Some descriptive statistics for questionnaires
Responsive	Interviews, naturalistic observation	Qualitative analysis

ACTIVITY 45

Read the following case study and then answer the questions that follow.

> **Cynthia** (the nursery nurse mentioned in the case study on page 89) evaluates a new mode of attendance of children at a day nursery by sending a questionnaire to all parents to see how satisfied they are with the new system. She also interviews each member of staff to find out what effect the new system has had on their working practices.
>
> The questionnaire comprises a series of dichotomous questions (yes/no). The staff interview is semi-structured with a series of open-ended questions designed to allow staff to express their feelings freely.
>
> The questionnaire data reveal that:
>
> ● 85 per cent of respondents prefer the new system to the old system
>
> ● of those respondents who prefer the new system, 90 per cent work full-time
>
> ● of the 15 per cent who prefer the old system 10 per cent work part-time and 5 per cent work shifts.
>
> Cynthia interviewed six members of staff using a tape-recorder. The key issues that emerged most frequently from the data were:
>
> ● disruption to the working routine (4 respondents) which caused
>
> ● difficulty in getting children to settle to routine.

1   What level of measurement was used in the questionnaire?

2   In what ways were descriptive statistics used in the questionnaire data?

3 State a hypothesis that could be formed from the questionnaire data. You may, for example, hypothesise that the number of respondents who answer in a certain way are also likely to have certain characteristics.

4 State the independent variable and the dependent variable for your hypothesis.

5 State the null hypothesis for your hypothesis.

6 Is the hypothesis one-tailed or two-tailed?

7 Which statistical test would be used to test this hypothesis? Give reasons for your answer.

8 What processes would Cynthia have used to arrive at the key issues derived from the interviews?

9 Write a paragraph summarising the findings of the interview data.

Commentary

1   The **nominal level** of measurement (yes/no) was used in the questionnaire, this being the simplest, least powerful level of measurement.

2   Descriptive statistics were used to describe the questionnaire data in the form of percentages.

3   A hypothesis that could be formed from the questionnaire results would be 'respondents who work full-time are more satisfied with the new system than respondents who work part-time or shifts.'

4   The independent variable in the hypothesis in (3) is the *type of work* and the dependent variable is *satisfaction with new system*. (Since you may have chosen a different hypothesis to ours, you should check your answers to questions 4-7 with a tutor.)

5   The null hypothesis here is 'there is no relationship between satisfaction with the new system of nursery attendance and parental working patterns'.

6   The hypothesis is one-tailed because the hypothesis states the *direction* of the expected change, in other words, that respondents will be *more* satisfied.

7   The statistical test that would be used to test this hypothesis is the Chi-square test. This is because this test is used to see whether there is a relationship between two or more variables (in this case 'working patterns' and 'satisfaction with new system'). The test relies on nominal data ('works full-time', 'does not work full-time' and 'satisfied/dissatisfied'). Two or more groups are required for this test to be used. In this case the parents can be divided into those who work full-time and those who work part-time or shifts.

8   Cynthia would have used the following processes to arrive at the key issues derived from the interviews:

   ● transcribing of the tapes (data display)

   ● developing categories and themes from the data through content analysis (data reduction).

9   The following summary could be made of the interview data:

   The new system causes some problems as well as some potential improvements. The problems highlighted most frequently were concerned with 'disruption of routine' which caused problems in trying to get children to settle. Not knowing when children were expected to arrive caused increased stress on staff. Despite these difficulties staff did perceive the new system as being more flexible and as creating better staff relationships with parents.

Nominal data: The simplest level of measurement in which dichotomous data can be categorised into two groupings such as male/female, yes/no, pass/fail.

The final activity will help you to apply what you have learned in this session to your own research.

ACTIVITY 46   ALLOW **15** MINUTES

Write down an area of your work in which you would like to carry out an evaluative study. (You may use an example from an earlier activity if you wish.) Then answer the questions below.

My evaluative study

1 Is your research summative or formative?

2 Is your research qualitative or quantitative or a combination of both?

3 Which of the five approaches to evaluative research would you use?

4 What would be your chosen methods of data collection?

5 How would you analyse the data? If inferential statistics are to be used, state which test you would use.

Commentary

Since it is obviously impossible for us to know what your particular response is, you should share your ideas with other students and seek the advice of a tutor or mentor to ensure that you are on the right track.

Summary

1 Through the process of clarifying your research study you will be aware of the need to carefully select the setting from which data are gleaned. In many cases, this will be the environment where care is delivered.

2 Important considerations about ethical approval for research proposals have been explored through the use of case study material.

3 The complexities of sampling have been discussed. The importance of selecting the most appropriate sample to match your research design has been established.

4 The essential differences between qualitative and quantitative evaluative data have been discussed, along with various methods of data collection.

5 You have been taken through the analysis of data and the type of statistics that can be generated depending on the research design used.

Before you move on to Session Six, check that you have achieved the objectives given at the beginning of this session and, if not, review the appropriate sections.

Using evaluative research to influence decision-making

Introduction

This session will build on the research project that you have designed in previous sessions by considering how to disseminate your findings so that they will actually impact on service provision. You will have the opportunity to read various research articles and answer questions on them. You will also learn about ways of disseminating research findings.

Session objectives

When you have completed this session you should be able to:

- understand research-based articles in the field of evaluative research
- plan strategies to disseminate your findings and influence service delivery
- prepare your findings from evaluative research as:
    - a written report
    - a journal article
    - a conference paper.

1: Reading evaluative research

Most research articles follow a similar format in terms of presentation.

- *An introduction* explains the background to the study and cites several studies on which the research is based. The research question or problem is also provided.

- *A methodology section* outlines the design of the study including sample selection and tools used to collect the data.

- *A results section* presents the main findings, often in the form of tables, graphs or histograms.

- *A discussion section* discusses the main findings and compares them with other studies.

- *A conclusion* summarises the main points and gives the main findings of the research.

When reading research articles it is important to be able to evaluate the article as well as the way in which the research was conducted and what the main findings were. The table below indicates the main points you will need to consider under each of the headings listed above.

Heading	Points to evaluate
Introduction	Is the research question or problem researchable?
	Is the research problem sufficiently important to justify the research?
	Is the background to the research relevant to the research question/s?
Methodology	Is the sample large enough to be representative of the wider population?
	Does the sampling strategy suggest that the research can be generalisable to other similar groups?
	Are the instruments used to collect data valid and reliable?
	Were the subjects harmed or inconvenienced in any way?
	Was the research designed in such a way that unwanted influences, such as gender or age, were controlled?
Results	Are the results presented in such a way that they can be understood?
	Were the results analysed appropriately?
Discussion	Did the researcher illuminate the most pertinent results?
	Were the results used to support or refute results of other studies?
	Did the discussion of the results successfully address the research question/s?

Conclusion	Did the conclusion successfully draw out the main points of the research?
	Did the conclusion suggest recommendations based on the research?
	Did the conclusion suggest areas for future research?

Not all articles are presented in exactly the way described above. However, you should still be able to extract the information in the table above from somewhere in the article. In the activities that follow we apply this approach to a series of articles.

ACTIVITY 47   ALLOW 30 MINUTES

Read *Resource 1* in the *Resources Section* and then answer the following questions.

1 What were the aims of Kent's study?

2 What methods of data collection were used?

3 What were the main findings in relation to shared learning? (The main findings are often conveyed within the paragraphs under the relevant sub-heading. Normally one or two key findings will be found in each paragraph.)

4 What were the main findings in relation to practice placements?

5 Were qualitative or quantitative methods used?

6 What approach to evaluation does this study most closely resemble?

7 Is the study an example of formative or summative evaluation?

8 Why can this study be described as an evaluative study?

Commentary

1 The purpose of Kent's study was to find out whether or not midwives need first to train as nurses by focusing specifically on two areas of the curricula: shared learning and nursing placements.

2 Methods used to collect data were:

- the use of six sites as case studies (chosen from 17 programmes available in England in 1991)

- documentary analysis of curricula and course documents

- a detailed group inquiry to explore student educational experiences at two sites.

3 The main findings in relation to shared learning were that:

- shared sessions were too biased towards nursing, giving too few midwifery examples

- there is little agreement between curriculum planners as to whether shared learning with nursing students is the best way of achieving a foundation knowledge early in the programme

- timetabling difficulties caused two courses to abandon shared learning

- the minority status of midwives caused isolation, although they themselves actually encouraged others to regard them as distinct from other students

- some midwifery teachers felt that alliances were politically expedient rather than being educationally led and this meant that the midwifery content was diluted

- assisting students to apply shared lectures to midwifery was time-consuming

- shared learning is cost-effective and prevents midwives becoming too insular.

4   The main findings in relation to practice placements were that:

- all pre-registration midwifery students were expected to spend some time in nursing areas

- in one case students spent most of their first year in nursing areas and this caused some frustration due to the time that elapsed before they could practise midwifery

- in cases where nursing placements occurred in the second year students felt de-skilled because they had just begun to gain confidence in midwifery skills

- the diversity of placements indicated different views about what is essential or useful in midwifery education

- nurses in some areas were inadequately prepared to be mentors and supervisors for student midwives and were confused by their presence

- some students carried out menial tasks and gained only a superficial view of nursing.

5   The use of interviews and the researcher's interpretation of the curriculum mean that the study uses a qualitative approach.

6   The evaluative approach which appears to be used for this study is the decision-focused approach. This is because the study is clearly a component of a national study commissioned by the Department of Health. The DoH would therefore probably agree the methodology to be used and require the researchers to produce regular reports of their progress.

7   Although Kent does not specify whether this is a summative or formative evaluation it corresponds most closely to a summative evaluation because of the large-scale nature of the evaluation and the requirement for a final summative report. It is also most unlikely that changes could be made during the evaluation (as would be typical of a formative evaluation study).

8   Although Kent does not describe her study as an evaluative study in her article, it could be so called because she is attempting to evaluate the effectiveness of something – shared learning and placements in midwifery education. Her analysis of her findings indicates a genuine desire to find out from the participants how useful the experiences of shared learning and placements are. The findings from this research, like all evaluative research, can be used to indicate where changes need to be made in the programme of study. In fact, Kent's findings make it quite explicit where changes need to be made to make shared learning and placements more effective.

ACTIVITY 48   ALLOW 45 MINUTES

Read *Resource 2* in the *Resources Section* and then answer the following questions.

1   What was the purpose of the study?

2   What methods of data collection were used?

3 Is this an example of qualitative or quantitative research?

4 What do the results show?

5 Which of the five approaches to evaluative research does this study most closely resemble?

6 Is the study an example of formative or summative evaluation?

7 What type of statistics were used?

8 Why can this study be described as evaluative research?

Commentary

1 The purpose of this study was to determine the appropriateness of referrals from primary care to secondary care.

2 An analysis of referral letters and the outcome of the referral was the chosen method. These records were evaluated independently by two doctors: the referring doctor and a doctor who had access to similar services. A questionnaire was used to determine whether each referral was avoidable or not.

3 This is an example of quantitative research because the questionnaire

comprised closed-ended questions. The results of the questionnaire could then be recorded in numerical form and subjected to statistical calculation.

4   The results showed that:

● in 34 per cent of cases referrals were avoidable

● most of this 34 per cent were referred due to a lack of resources

● many of the 26 avoidable referrals that were due to limitations of knowledge could have been avoided in a group practice because the GP could have sought a second opinion from a colleague.

5   This is a difficult question to answer because the study does not really resemble any of the approaches. The concerns of service users were not addressed as would be typical of a user-orientated or responsive approach; nor were decision-makers involved, as would be typical of a decision-focused approach. It probably most closely resembles the goal-orientated approach if we can assume that the goals of general practice are:

● to refer patients for secondary care as appropriate

● to initiate the use of secondary care resources in primary health care.

The use of quantitative methods are typical of the goal-orientated approach.

6   The research has elements of both formative and summative evaluation. It is typical of formative research because of its small-scale and local nature. However, because the data were collected retrospectively it was not possible to make changes to the service during the data collection phase. This is more typical of summative research (in which a report is produced at the end of the study).

7   The research uses descriptive statistics which can be presented in tabular form and as percentages.

8   The research can be described as evaluative because the results can be used to improve service provision. In particular, the results could be used to demonstrate the need for additional resources in the primary healthcare sector in order to reduce the number of avoidable referrals and save money. This GP has shown, through evaluating the effectiveness of his referrals, that his performance is ineffective because of a lack of supportive resources.

ACTIVITY 49
ALLOW 45 MINUTES

Read *Resource 3* in the *Resources Section* and then answer the following questions.

1   What was the purpose of the study?

2   What methods of data collection were used?

3   Is this an example of qualitative or quantitative research?

4   What did the results show?

5   Which of the five approaches to evaluative research most closely resembles this study?

6   Is the study an example of formative or summative evaluation?

7   What type of statistics were used?

8   Why can this study be described as evaluative research?

Commentary

1   The purpose of the study was to evaluate primary nursing in a nursing development unit, and to validate or reject the previous subjective evaluation. Primary nursing is an organised approach to care in which each nurse (the 'named nurse') is responsible for the care of a small group of patients. The researcher was particularly interested in whether interactions were mainly conducted on an individual basis (primary), with a small group (team), or with any nurse from a ward (task allocation).

2   The study used a previously validated audit tool which is a classification system for clarification, understanding and measurement of nurses' work

methods. It is described as a 'work method assessment sheet' which has structured components scored according to the results of interviews with nurses and patients. The interviews are carried out by the auditor who then allocates a score on the sheet according to the responses of the interviewees.

3   This is an example of quantitative research (even though interviews are used) because of the allocation of numerical scores which can be counted.

4   The results show that:

●   the scores indicated the use of team nursing, rather than primary nursing or task allocation

●   there was a discrepancy between the auditor's perception of how the nurses work was organised and how it actually was

●   the result was disappointing but could have been affected by structural and organisational changes at the time of the audit

●   the tool was easy to use

●   the tool assisted in clarifying, classifying, understanding and measuring organisation of nursing care.

5   The approach to evaluative research could be described as goal-orientated because the goals of primary nursing, although not clearly specified in the article, underpinned the study.

6   The study is an example of formative evaluation because the evaluation is an ongoing process – further evaluation was planned.

7   Descriptive statistics were used which were presented as raw scores in the article.

8   The study can be described as evaluative research because of a stated wish to use the findings to improve the delivery of services.

ACTIVITY 50   ALLOW 45 MINUTES

Read *Resource 4* in the *Resources Section* and then answer the following questions.

1   What was the purpose of the study?

2   List three justifications used by the authors for combining qualitative and quantitative methods.

3   Why was a qualitative study used to develop further what had already been discovered using quantitative analysis?

4 Which of the five approaches to evaluative research was used for this study?

5 What type of data analysis was used?

6 Why can this study be described as evaluative research?

Commentary

1 The purpose of the study was to determine whether generic problems in health delivery existed in some areas of Colorado and to assess the perception of solutions to these problems from the communities that experienced them.

2 The following justifications were given for combining qualitative and quantitative methods:

- each method can be used to explain the results obtained from the other method

- qualitative methods can be used as the basis for the development of quantitative methods

- the two methods can be used to cross-validate findings, thus strengthening confidence in the results.

3 Quantitative data revealed that there was no significant difference between the rural and urban areas of America in relation to preventable cancers, thereby suggesting that access to care was also similar. The authors believed that the real problems in rural Colorado communities were not reflected in the data and therefore superimposed a qualitative study on to quantitative findings in order to provide a broader picture of health service delivery in these areas.

4 A user-orientated approach was the approach taken in this study because the researchers sought the views of a variety of different key informants, including influential people, health care workers and service users.

5 The results were analysed using qualitative analysis. Three categories were first identified and the interview transcripts were then classified accordingly. Data were then tallied according to the type of interviewee.

6 The use of the research findings to identify solutions to the problems identified makes this a good example of evaluative research.

You probably found that the articles you read in these activities used slightly different approaches to presenting research findings. Nevertheless, they do all explain to the reader the nature of the research, its background, the way in which it was conducted and the findings. We will now consider how well-presented research findings can influence policy makers.

2: Evaluation and the policy process

There is little point in going to the trouble of carrying out evaluative research if the results are not going to be considered by policy makers. As discussed in Session One, the purpose of evaluative research is to evaluate the effectiveness of a programme in order to determine whether any changes need to be made or whether the programme should be withdrawn. We discussed how the implications of this can be threatening for people who don't want their faults exposed. We also saw how this threat can extend to policy-makers, who may know that they have an obligation to evaluate their services, but who don't have the resources to make any amendments that might be recommended by the researcher.

When planning your research, then, you will need to take the needs of policy and decision-makers into consideration and gain their co-operation before you commence your study.

One writer who is particularly concerned about the impact of evaluative research on policy-makers is Hailey (1992). Hailey raises some important points which are explored in the next activity.

ACTIVITY 51   ALLOW 35 MINUTES

Read the chapter by Hailey in *Resource 5* in the *Resources Section* and then answer the questions below.

1   What does Hailey see as the main problems with evaluative research's capacity to influence policy?

2   What is one solution that he sees to the problem?

3   What are the most prevalent attitudes of policy-makers towards evaluative research according to Hailey?

4   What are the particular problems with evaluating preventive health care which Hailey identifies?

Commentary

1   Hailey believes that evaluative data cannot easily be assimilated into policy decisions and can even be considered embarrassing if they point to major flaws in service provision. He warns that 'the most elegant and detailed analysis may have no impact on the policy process if:

   ● the timing is wrong

   ● the results are not presented in a way that is intelligible to policy makers

   ● the recommendations are unrealistic in political terms.'

2   Hailey's solution is for evaluators to continue their efforts to communicate with policy-makers, to describe their health care programmes clearly so that they are comprehensible to policy advisers and to provide intelligible and quick analysis.

3   The attitudes of policy-makers towards evaluative research which Hailey discusses include the views that:

   ● it helps the health authority to push away the problem – deferring decision-making

   ● consultants are useful in that they can generate quick opinions which can be accepted or rejected with no one else involved

   ● lack of control over evaluators is a problem.

4   The problem Hailey identifies is that, while evaluation may be lengthy and require long-term protocols, policy-makers and governments want to see a quick return on expenditure.

We can see from the above activity that evaluative research does have its problems and that you will need to work closely with decision-makers when carrying it out. You will need to:

● conduct your research in a manner that is convenient to decision-makers, whilst recognising that it may take considerable time to collect data

● produce a timely and clear written report which is sufficiently brief and clear that it will have an immediate impact upon decision-makers.

Now that we have established the need to co-operate with decision-makers and to produce a timely and clear written report, we will go on to discuss the dissemination of your findings in more detail.

3: Disseminating your findings

There are several ways you can disseminate your research findings. The most important are in:

- written reports

- journal articles

- conference papers.

We will now look at each of these in turn.

Presenting a research report

A written report is the most suitable means to use when presenting your findings to decision-makers. We have already considered the importance of making reports brief and clear so that busy managers can read them quickly. Although your full research report will probably be well over 5,000 words in length, an edited version of no more than 2,000 would be more suitable for decision-makers.

It is important that you fully understand the conventions for the organisation and presentation of research reports. First, it should always be written in the past tense. This is because it explains the nature of the study you conducted, why you did it and how you did it. Second, it is important to allow appropriate 'weighting' to the different components of the report. As a general rule, the introduction should use about 10 per cent of the words of the entire report and the conclusion should use another 10 per cent of the words. The review of the literature should use about 20 per cent of the words and the remaining 60 per cent should be equally divided between the methodology section, the discussion and the results.

The third point to bear in mind when writing your research report is to write very *specifically* about what you actually did, rather than discussing theories and research methods in an abstract manner.

Fourth, you should use sub-headings to guide your reader through your research study. You should formulate paragraphs under each sub-heading so that each paragraph addresses a specific issue.

Finally, your research will need to be clearly referenced to the theories and research on which it is based. You will need to check with your tutor which referencing system is appropriate for your work. In most cases this is the Harvard system, but the Vancouver system is also frequently used.

ACTIVITY 52	ALLOW 15 MINUTES

A breakdown of the contents of a research report is reproduced in *Figure 14*. Using a separate sheet of paper, review these contents in relation to your own evaluative research study which you have used in previous activities in this unit. Consider how you will apply the headings to your own study.

Contents of a research report

- *Title* should include very specific *key words* which would be used by students conducting a CD-ROM search when attempting to research a similar area.

- *Abstract*, describing in approximately 100 words the research problem, methods and findings of the study. This would be written in the past tense, explaining very briefly what you did and what you found.

- *Introduction*, to include:

  a statement of the research problem

  background to the study

  any theories on which the study is based

  any research questions or hypotheses that guide the study

  definitions of relevant terms used in the question or hypothesis.

- *Brief account of the literature* pertaining to the subject.

- *Methodology*, to include:

  sample selection

  attempts made to control the research, including extraneous variables

  description of data-collection instruments, with a rationale for their use and details about how they were developed

  procedures undertaken in actual collection of data, including the logistics of how and when questionnaires were distributed or how exactly interviews or observations were carried out.

- *Presentation and analysis of data*, in which tables are accurately presented (unless qualitative data is used), labelled and discussed within the text.

- *Discussion* of the main findings of the study, including how they related to similar previous findings, the extent to which they are generalisable to other populations and their implications for practice.

- *Conclusion and recommendations*, indicating the overall findings from the study, how they relate to the research problem, question or hypothesis, and any recommendations for future service delivery.

Figure 14: An example of how to break down the contents of a research report

Commentary

Your response to this activity will obviously be very personal to your own sphere of practice. It would be useful at this stage to discuss your research with a tutor to ensure that you are on the right lines.

Writing articles for journals

Journal articles are always an excellent way to disseminate your research findings. They allow you to share your work with a much greater number of people than would otherwise be the case. Before writing an evaluative report for publication, you need to contact the relevant decision-makers to make sure that they are willing for the results to be published. You also need to be absolutely sure that the specific situation in which the research was carried out cannot be identified by readers. If your research is critical of service provision, the decision-makers concerned may not wish the results to be published even if the details are anonymous. On the other hand, your research findings may show a high quality of service provision which decision-makers will be only too happy to share with others and you may therefore be actively encouraged to publish your findings.

If you are successful in requesting permission from decision-makers to publish your findings then you will need to think about the content of your article. Articles are normally shorter than research reports – often about 3,000 words. You will need to select a suitable journal and find out the protocol for submission of articles for publication. You will need to follow the specific guidelines carefully. Generally, the guidance in *Figure 14* for writing research reports also applies to journal articles. Once you have selected a journal it is a good idea to skim read some of the articles to gain a sense of the types of headings used and the style and quality of article published. For example, some journals target senior managers or academics whilst others are designed for practitioners.

Getting articles published is a competitive business because there is a limited amount of journal space and an increasing number of practitioners in health and social care who have produced work worthy of publication. Don't be deterred if your article is not accepted for publication by the first journal you approach. Journal editorial panels have different priorities and some themes are more important to them at particular times. You will also need to be patient when waiting to find out whether your article is accepted for publication because some panels take several months to reach a decision.

Preparing conference papers

Conference papers are similar to published articles in that they enable you to share your findings with a large number of people. However, at conferences you also have a valuable opportunity for dialogue with the people on the receiving end of your presentation. This means that you can share ideas with them for the further development of your research.

It is not too difficult to avail yourself of opportunities to speak at conferences. If you decide you want to speak at conferences you will need to read regular bulletins in journals to keep informed of possible occasions on which to present your findings. Conference organisers normally send out a 'call for papers' bulletin about nine months before the conference. These are often sent to managers but may also appear as 'flyers' in popular journals such as the *Nursing Times*.

Conferences are also advertised in journals and the advertisements also often include calls for papers. These inform potential speakers of the type of subjects that are applicable to the conference as well as the required format for the presentation of an abstract. Interested speakers complete the relevant form and send a summary of their research, usually no more than 200 words.

If your paper were to be accepted you would then prepare a more detailed report for presentation, as well as any audio visual aids such as over-head transparencies or slides. As with journal publications, you would need to gain permission from decision-makers before presenting your findings at a conference, and again ensure that the specific situation from which the data are acquired cannot be identified.

A final activity will help you to consider how best you could disseminate the findings of your research.

ACTIVITY 53   ALLOW **10** MINUTES

Return once again to the research that you have used in previous activities and think about the following questions.

		YES	NO
1	Do you intend to produce a written report?	☐	☐
2	If yes, have you discussed the nature of your written report with a tutor?	☐	☐
3	Are you interested in publishing your findings in a journal?	☐	☐
4	If yes, have you decided which journal is appropriate?	☐	☐
5	Are you interested in presenting your findings at conferences?	☐	☐
6	If yes, have you found out about any relevant forthcoming conferences?	☐	☐

Commentary

We hope that you will have answered 'yes' to some of these questions! Don't forget: you must gain permission from decision-makers before publishing your results in journals or speaking at conferences.

Summary

1   This session has used a number of articles to help you get used to making practical sense of evaluative research. We have also discussed ways in which you can prepare and report your research findings both locally and nationally.

2   We have seen how research reports can influence the quality of service delivery.

We hope you have found this unit useful in helping you to apply the knowledge you have gained from other units in this series to evaluative research. By now, you should feel more confident in reading and understanding research articles and should be thinking about your own data collection and ways you can use this to influence and improve service provision. Don't worry if you found that you had forgotten some of the earlier units before embarking on this one. Research is a subject which involves referring frequently to text books before embarking on a study. This unit and other units in this series will act as reference sources at different stages of your study.

LEARNING REVIEW

Before you started work on this unit, you were asked to complete a learning profile to assess your current level of knowledge and identify key areas on which you particularly needed to focus. Now that you have completed the unit, use the list of anticipated outcomes to review the progress you have made during your study of evaluative research methodology. These are repeated below.

For each outcome, tick the box that most closely corresponds to the point you feel you have now reached and compare it with your response in the Learning Profile. If there are any areas that you still find difficult to understand, you should find it helpful to review the sessions concerned and to discuss any remaining problems with your tutor.

	Not at all	Partly	Quite well	Very well

Session One

I can:

- define evaluative research ☐ ☐ ☐ ☐

- outline the purpose of evaluative research ☐ ☐ ☐ ☐

- distinguish between evaluative research and exploratory research ☐ ☐ ☐ ☐

- explain the use of evaluative research as an example of critical research methodology ☐ ☐ ☐ ☐

- discuss how evaluative research can be used to influence policy formation and decision making. ☐ ☐ ☐ ☐

Session Two

I can:

- recall the meaning of qualitative and quantitative research ☐ ☐ ☐ ☐

- describe the 'black box' and give examples of the methods of data collection used for each approach to evaluative research ☐ ☐ ☐ ☐

- explain inductive and deductive approaches to theory development in evaluative research ☐ ☐ ☐ ☐

- define the meaning of triangulation as it applies to evaluative research. ☐ ☐ ☐ ☐

	Not at all	Partly	Quite well	Very well

Session Three

I can:

- distinguish between formative and summative designs in evaluative research ☐ ☐ ☐ ☐

- distinguish between experimental and quasi-experimental design in evaluative research ☐ ☐ ☐ ☐

- understand the notations used in experimental and quasi-experimental designs ☐ ☐ ☐ ☐

- explain how to design an evaluative research study to establish the value of a programme. ☐ ☐ ☐ ☐

Session Four

I can:

- describe the advantages and disadvantages of the following approaches to evaluative research:

  experimental ☐ ☐ ☐ ☐

  goal-orientated ☐ ☐ ☐ ☐

  decision-focused ☐ ☐ ☐ ☐

  user-orientated ☐ ☐ ☐ ☐

  responsive ☐ ☐ ☐ ☐

- describe why the responsive approach is an example of critical research methodology. ☐ ☐ ☐ ☐

Session Five

I can:

- plan how to gain access to relevant settings for data collection purposes ☐ ☐ ☐ ☐

- select and justify a choice of sampling frame for data collection ☐ ☐ ☐ ☐

- design questionnaires and interview schedules appropriately ☐ ☐ ☐ ☐

	Not at all	Partly	Quite well	Very well

Session Five *continued*

- use descriptive and inferential statistics to analyse survey data from evaluative research □ □ □ □

- recall how to use qualitative data analysis to analyse open-ended responses and observations derived from evaluative research. □ □ □ □

Session Six

I can:

- understand research-based articles in the field of evaluative research □ □ □ □

- plan strategies to disseminate research findings and influence service delivery □ □ □ □

- prepare findings from evaluative research as:

  a written report □ □ □ □

  a journal article □ □ □ □

  a conference paper. □ □ □ □

RESOURCES SECTION

Contents

RESOURCE 1

*From Nursing Times
(June 14, Vol.91, No.24,
1995)*

Evaluating pre-registration midwifery education

Key words

Pre-registration midwifery education, research, shared learning, midwifery.

Abstract

This paper examines the findings of a Department of Health-funded evaluation of pre-registration midwifery education in England and explores whether there is any need for midwives to train first as nurses. The research was completed in 1993 and this paper accepted for publication in January 1994.

Julie Kent, BSc, RGN, was research associate for Maggs Research Associates when she carried out this evaluation project, funded by the DoH. She is now lecturer in sociology at the University of the West of England, Bristol.

In 1990 the Department of Health funded a three-year evaluation of pre-registration midwifery education in England.[1] Sixteen sites where pre-registration midwifery education (Box 1) was provided agreed to take part in the evaluation. This included all 17 programmes that were current in October 1991[2] and two additional programmes that began at the same sites after this date.

Six of these sites were also selected as case studies.[3] Semi-structured interviews with midwife teachers, student midwives, midwifery managers, midwife mentors, non-midwife teachers and obstetricians took place at these sites. In addition, I carried out documentary analysis of curricula and course documents. A detailed 'group inquiry' also explored the students' educational experiences at two sites.[4]

This paper refers to these data as part of a national picture, and examines whether midwives need to train first as nurses. It focuses specifically on two areas of the curricula: shared learning and nursing placements. These may be seen as critical to ensuring that midwives trained via the pre-registration route develop the 'nursing skills' necessary to care for women who, for example, have pregnancies complicated by epilepsy, diabetes or cardiac anomalies, or assumed to be necessary because the majority of women are hospitalised for their delivery.[5]

Of the 19 programmes included in the evaluation, six diploma programmes were found to have no shared learning, nine had shared learning with nurses on Project 2000 courses; three degree programmes had shared learning with nursing degree students and three had some shared learning with other students in higher education (Box 2). On one of these, student midwives had shared learning with medical and dental students.

Shared learning

Shared learning is usually in the biological and social sciences, although it may include professional studies or study and research skills (Box 2). Commonly, non-midwife

---

Box 1. The pre-registration approach to midwifery education

Since 1989 there has been a mushrooming of courses enabling people to train as a midwife without first training as a nurse. Once referred to as 'direct entry', but now termed pre-registration midwifery programmes, these are open to those who are not already registered on Parts 1 or 12 of the UKCC register.

By June 1993 there were 35 validated pre-registration midwifery programmes in England. Of these, seven are degree programmes and the remainder are at diploma level. Most programmes are of three years duration but five of the degree programmes are four-year courses. The growth in the number of programmes has exceeded the Department of Health's expectations since it provided pump-priming funds for 14 sites in 1989-90 and 1990-91 as part of its 'policy of support' for pre-registration midwifery education.

teachers take these shared sessions and they are either specialist subject teachers from an institution of higher education (such as a university) or nurse teachers from a college of nursing and midwifery. Generally, midwife teachers did not teach mixed student groups. The amount of shared learning is difficult to quantify, but it took place during the first year or 18 months of a programme. Students often criticised the content of these shared sessions for being too biased towards nursing, giving too few midwifery examples and having little relevance for them.[6] Some non-midwife teachers recognised that they cater mainly for a group of nurses and that on occasion it is difficult to meet the needs of midwifery students.

Curriculum planners argue there is a need for 'foundation knowledge' in the early part of the programme. However, there is little agreement as to whether shared sessions with nursing students are the best means of achieving this. In one case, shared learning was set up with medical and dental students in the hope that better understanding between doctors and midwives might follow. This was, however, later dropped and replaced by shared teaching with biology students, as the content of lectures was found to be inappropriate. In two cases no shared learning had developed. This was partly because of timetabling difficulties in one, although in the other there was little enthusiasm for shared learning.

The small numbers of student midwives on most programmes (10-25) compounded their minority status in large teaching groups. Isolation characterised their experience although, paradoxically, they often encouraged others to regard them as distinct from other students. Where they were taught with medical students they felt their age and gen-

der set them apart.

Many midwife teachers recognised that political and organisational factors had shaped the way shared learning had developed. Even though midwives had rejected the idea that midwifery was a branch of nursing during consultations with the UKCC over Project 2000,[7,8] they found that associations with nursing courses were a matter of political expedience and appeared necessary if midwifery were to survive at all in some institutions. The alliances that developed, therefore, were not always educationally led and some felt the midwifery content of programmes had been diluted as a result.[9] The teaching of midwifery topics was sometimes determined by the programme for shared learning and did not necessarily follow any logic in midwifery terms. Other midwife teachers spent their time assisting students to apply the shared lectures to midwifery, which was time-consuming, and had to supplement the teaching by the specialist teacher. Historically, this had been common practice in nurse education.[10] The two main arguments in support of shared learning are that it is cost-effective and prevents midwives from becoming too insular. While at first sight it appears that it does rationalise resources, if midwife teachers spend time elaborating on key lectures and, in effect, repeating material, then resources and time are being wasted. The second argument is difficult to sustain since so many midwives and others remarked on the ways that midwifery students stood out within larger student groups. Points of difference were highlighted rather than common interests identified and students themselves sought to emphasise their identity as midwives.

Finally, there is little to suggest that shared learning brings any other benefits. In edu-

---

Box 2. Shared learning

Shared learning refers to arrangements where students from more than one course attend the same lectures or seminars. Normally, it takes the form of 'key lectures' attended by a large group of students and is one way institutions may rationalise teaching resources. It is also argued that such sessions provide an opportunity to develop and enhance relationships between student groups and so promote better interprofessional relations.

The rationale for shared learning includes ideas about the knowledge and skills that may be common to students on different courses.

The ENB encourages shared learning, which it defines as 'a planned approach or strategy within a curriculum leading to sharing of knowledge and experience between groups'. The board considers it desirable to 'take advantage of common modules with other courses...where appropriate'.[14]

cational terms there was little agreement about what might usefully constitute a 'common module' or 'foundation knowledge'. Instead, there was widespread dissatisfaction with the content and timing of shared learning. Those who had experienced it had little enthusiasm for developing it further and often would have preferred less.

However, views about the value of shared learning raise fundamental questions about the kind of knowledge and skills a midwife needs. Downe[11] argues that any suggestion that midwifery courses should increase links with Project 2000 nursing programmes could lend credence to the view that midwifery should, or will, after all become a branch of nursing. According to her, this should be resisted.

Placements in nursing area

Differing terminology points to underlying ambivalence about the purpose and value of 'nursing', 'specialist' or 'non-midwifery' placements. For some midwife teachers these placements were based on the belief that midwives need to develop certain 'nursing skills', for others they afford an opportunity to develop what are essentially midwifery skills in 'specialist' areas.

All pre-registration midwifery students were expected to spend time in nursing areas although the pattern and length of placements varied between programmes. The first placement offered included short observation visits with the primary health-care team, but most students spent more time with the community midwife. In some cases this was part of an introduction to a health care or common core programme. In one case students spent much of their first year in nursing areas, including an orthopaedic, medical or surgical ward, chest unit or psychiatric unit. In this case, individual students had quite different placements, that were centrally allocated and took no account of their status as midwifery students. The placements were related to common modules in the first 18 months of the programme and although the students gained some experience of community midwifery, they had no hospital midwifery experience until the end of the second year of the four-year programme. Students were frustrated by the amount of time spent in these areas and the length of time that elapsed before they were able to focus on midwifery.

In other cases, placements in nursing areas were in the second year of three-year programmes. This led students to feel deskilled at a time when they had just begun to gain confidence in their midwifery skills.

From the curriculum analysis of the six case studies, placements included paediatric units, medical and mental health or psychiatry units, special care and neonatal units, and learning disability services.

The diversity of placements between courses points to a range of views about what is regarded as an essential or useful part of midwifery education, and was the product of divergent educational philosophies and/or the facilities available locally. Indeed, students on the same programme could have very different experiences if they were placed at different hospital sites in that area.

However, the content of placements was heavily criticised. Staff were described as being unfamiliar with the pre-registration midwifery programme and having little understanding of midwifery. They were said to have been puzzled by the presence of midwifery students in these areas and, while midwife mentors had been prepared for the new programmes, there was no evidence that nurses in these areas had been prepared to act as mentors or supervisors to pre-registration midwifery students. One group of students felt they had learnt some useful skills, such as caring for a patient with intravenous infusion and giving injections, but they also said that much time had been spent carrying out 'menial tasks' and they had gained only a very superficial view of nursing during that time.

Midwife teachers recognised that there had been difficulties but did not always agree with students that the placements had no value. Their views varied depending on whether they saw the placements as opportunities to develop essential 'nursing skills' or 'midwifery skills in a specialist area'.

However others, especially students, argued these skills could be taught in midwifery settings. The contractual relationships for purchasing and providing a programme have had increasing importance in shaping the organisation and administration of placements.

While some questioned how much experience of 'nursing' student midwives might need, few questioned the value of students spending time in midwifery areas, even though this seemed to add to the pressure of placing midwifery students elsewhere. The apparent overlap of nursing and midwifery curricula, like the shared learning discussion above, is a manifestation of a continuing association between the two professions, which remains ambiguous and controversial.

Conclusion

Among the midwives interviewed there was widespread agreement that they did not need to be a nurse to become a midwife. There was less agreement about what should be included in these programmes and about the value of either shared learning or placements in nursing areas.

> **Box 3. An agenda for midwifery education**
>
> The Association of Radical Midwives proposed that midwifery training should be primarily by a three-year direct entry course [15] and has suggested subjects to include in the curricula, as have some other writers.[16]
>
> The government supports the extension of pre-registration midwifery programmes and the expanding number of programmes suggests that pre-registration midwifery education is here to stay.[17]
>
> It has been argued that such programmes are more likely to promote a health-focused, holistic approach to midwifery care, that rejects a 'sickness' or 'ill health' model. In addition, midwives prepared in this way are expected to be better equipped to work more autonomously and be less willing to conform to hierarchical relationships.

Overall, there appeared to be an optimism that pre-registration midwifery programmes would strengthen the profession and improve standards of midwifery practice and that midwives thus trained would be agents of change. The evidence of the six case studies and the issues raised by those who took part in this evaluation suggest that current thinking continues to emphasise similarities between midwifery and nursing curricula and the importance of acquiring skills to care for women in hospital.

Organisational considerations have become confused with educational issues. It may be that the recommendations in Changing Childbirth[12] requiring providers of maternity services 'to demonstrate a significant shift towards a more community-orientated service' will encourage midwife teachers and education and service managers to re-examine the best means of contributing towards the development of such a service.

The claims of Project 2000 nursing courses to have a health focus and the move to a college-based education may mark an increasingly common base that midwifery and nursing students could usefully share. As we have seen, much would depend on the content and organisation of those sessions.[1]

The question that urgently needs to be addressed is: what does a woman need a midwife for? Answers to this question are primarily political, as the Expert Committee and House of Commons Health Committee reports have demonstrated.[12,13] But the answers will have consequences for education. If community midwifery services are to increase, a decrease in the amount of hospital-based midwifery training may be appropriate (Box 3). Changes in the division of labour between midwives, doctors and other health professionals and a redrawing of professional boundaries may have additional implications. The significance for midwifery education has yet to be fully worked out but a review of shared learning and placements in nursing areas is one place to start.

References

1 Kent, J., MacKeith, N., Maggs, C. *Direct But Different. An evaluation of pre-registration midwifery in England: A Research Project for the Department of Health.* London: DoH, 1994.

2 Kent, J., Maggs, C. *An Evaluation of Pre-Registration Midwifery in England: A Research Project for the Department of Health, Working Paper 1.* Research Design. Bath: Maggs Research Associates, 1992.

3 Kent, J. An evaluation of pre-registration midwifery in England. Research design: a case study approach. *Midwifery* 1992; 8: 69-75.

4 Kent, J. *With Women: A reflexive project.* PhD thesis. University of Bristol, 1995.

5 Downe, S. Dispelling the myths on direct entry training. *Nursing Times* 1986; 82: 37, 63-64.

6 Cardale, P. The direct route. *Nursing Times* 1992; 88: 13, 58-60.

7 UKCC *A New Preparation for Practice.* London: UKCC, 1986.

8 UKCC *P2000 and the Midwife.* London: UKCC, 1986.

9 Ho, E. Who is controlling midwifery education? *Midwifery Matters* 1991; 60: 24.

10 Maggs, C. *The Origins of General Nursing.* London: Croom Helm, 1983.

11 Downe, S. Midwives stand alone. *Nursing Times* 1990; 86: 24,22.

12 Department of Health, *Changing Childbirth.* London: HMSO, 1993.

13 House of Commons Health Committee. *Second Report on Maternity Services.* London: HMSO, 1992.

14 English National Board. *Regulations and Guidelines for Approval of Institutions*

and Courses. London: ENB, 1993.
15 Association of Radical Midwives. *The Vision: Proposals for the Future of the Maternity Services.* Osmirk: ARM, 1986.
16 Radford, N., Thompson, A. *Direct Entry: A preparation for midwifery practice.* Guildford: English National Board.

University of Surrey, 1988.
17 Department of Health. *Working for Patients: Education and training.* Working paper 10. London: HMSO, 1989.

RESOURCE 2

British Medical Journal,
(Vol. 309, pp 576-578)

Avoidable referrals? Analysis of 170 consecutive referrals to secondary care

Correspondence to: Dr Jones Elwyn.

Abstract

Objective – To determine appropriateness of referrals from primary care to secondary care.

Design – Retrospective evaluation of appropriateness of referrals from a singlehanded general practice: evaluations carried out independently by referring doctor and by second general practitioner who worked in same area and had access to similar secondary care services.

Subjects – 168 referrals made between 1 October 1990 and 31 March 1991 and followed up for up to 12 months by matching with available information on outcome of episode of care.

Main outcome measures – Appropriateness of referral and reasons for inappropriate referrals.

Results – 110 referrals were agreed to be appropriate and 58 were considered avoidable. The reason for 32 of the inappropriate referrals was lack of resources: 10 were due to lack of information (mainly failure of hospitals to pass on information to general practitioner), nine were due to a deficient primary health care team, five were due to insufficient use of home care nurses, three were due to absence of direct access to day hospital and five were due to lack of access to general practitioner beds or other facilities. Most of the remaining 26 avoidable referrals were because available resources had not been fully used, because recognised management plans had not been followed, or because of lack of skills to perform certain procedures.

Conclusions – Many theoretically avoidable referrals were due to managers' and politicians' decisions about allocation of resources, but some inappropriate referrals could be avoided by assessment of general practitioners' needs for further knowledge and skills.

Introduction

Referral rates for general practitioners vary widely even among doctors working in the same environment. Satisfactory explanations for such variation are elusive, even when medical education, sociodemographic features, morbidity and deprivation indices are controlled for.[1] It appears that general practitioners exhibit wide individual variation, which can be partly explained by chance[2] and partly by context and individual approaches to health care.

What is appropriate health care? What is an appropriate referral? These are complex questions that are viewed from differing perspectives by health care professionals, individual members of the public and society as a whole. There is a difference between appropriateness at the population level, which is always constrained by resources, and at an individual level, which is modified by the patient's characteristics and preferences or values.[4] The interplay of doctor, patient, illness and context is well understood in family medicine, where individual diagnosis is only one facet of clinical understanding.[5] It therefore comes as little surprise that variation in referral rates among general practitioners in Cambridge could not be explained by inappropriate referrals and that guide-lines would have made little difference.[6]

This study is the result of a singlehanded general practitioner's wish to determine whether any of his referrals could be deemed avoidable and what the reasons were for such referrals. The study is pragmatic in that it relates to the clinical realities in a singlehanded practice, where the context is as important as the content.

Questionnaire for audit of referrals

Name of patient: [ ]

Audit No: [ ]

Date of referral: [ ]

Speciality: [ ]

Prime instigator of referral:

General practitioner [ ]

Patient [ ]

Other (specify) [ ]

Not clear [ ]

Prime motive for referral:

For diagnosis [ ]

For opinion [ ]

For investigation [ ]

For management [ ]

For appliance [ ]

For 'breathing space' [ ]

For other opinion [ ]

Not clear [ ]

Time before patient seen at outpatient
department (to nearest No. of weeks): [ ]

If patient's notes not available:

Not currently registered [ ]

Dead [ ]

Seen as temporary patient [ ]

Outcome of process:

Patient not yet seen [ ]

Patient seen with good outcome [ ]

Patient seen with mediocre outcome [ ]

Patient seen with poor outcome [ ]

Could referral have been avoided and if so how?[†]

● No – appropriate referral for following reasons:

Need for specialist skills or procedure [ ]

Need for specialist knowledge [ ]

Need for specialist tests [ ]

Need for other perspective or opinion [ ]

● Yes – problem could have been managed in primary care if:

Doctor had more skills [ ]

Doctor had more knowledge [ ]

Doctor showed different attitude [ ]

Doctor had access to other resources [ ]

● Comment (how problems could have been managed in primary care):

● Appropriate benefit to patient or general practitioner with good
communication and appropriate follow up. [ ]

[†]To be completed by both evaluators.

Method

Copies were made of all referral letters sent from a singlehanded practice between 1 October 1990 and 31 March 1991. The practice consisted of 1800 patients, mainly of low socio-economic status living in a multi-ethnic inner city area. Patients' medical records were searched for the outcome of the referral: any correspondence from outpatient departments or hospital discharge letters were copied and linked with the original referral letter until the episode of care was completed or for up to 12 months after referral. Some records were not available because patients had died (18) or had registered elsewhere (five); it was not necessary to search for these records because the aim of the study was to focus on the reasons for any avoidable referrals rather than the rates of referral.

The referrals were evaluated independently by the referring doctor (GJE) and by a second doctor who worked in the same locality and had access to similar secondary care services (NCHS). Evaluations were made with an agreed questionnaire (see box), and the second doctor's role was to be as questioning as possible. The study's design meant that decisions were weighted towards classifying referrals as avoidable because the critical judgements were made when the outcome of each referral was available.

Results

In the six months of the study 170 referrals had been made. The general practitioner had been the prime instigator of 167 of the referrals, and patients had played a substantial role as co-instigators of 13 of the referrals. Assistance with management was requested in 159 cases, and diagnostic help was requested in 64. One referral was for an appliance, and one was to provide a 'breathing space' for the general practitioner. Waiting times varied greatly between specialist departments, but the average waiting time was 9-6 weeks. Fifteen patients did not attend their outpatient appointment.

Two referrals were excluded from the study because the second evaluator (NCHS) thought that there was insufficient information on which to base a judgement. In 124 of the remaining 168 cases we independently agreed on the appropriateness of referral. In 44 cases we discussed the independent evaluations and reached agreement: in 32 cases the referring doctor changed his categorisation to agree with the second evaluator (NCHS), and in 12 cases the second evaluator changed categorisation when context sensitive information was provided. We both felt that this process of discussing and agreeing categorisation was a valuable educational exercise.

The table summarises the evaluation of the referrals: 110 were agreed to be appropriate, and 58 were considered avoidable. Of the 32 inappropriate referrals that were considered to be due to lack of resources, 10 were because of a lack of information (mainly the failure of hospitals to pass on information to the general practitioner about a previous referral or contact); nine were due to a deficient primary health care team (mainly the lack of a community psychiatric nurse, but the lack of a health visitor and a dietician accounted for one referral each); five were due to insufficient use of home care nurses (leading to premature involvement of a palliative care consultant); and eight were due to lack of direct access to facilities (day hospital (three referrals) general practitioner beds (two referrals), and other facilities (three referrals)).

The general practitioner's attitude contributed to 12 avoidable referrals. In most of these cases available resources had not been used. In two cases hypertension that required further control was not managed to its full extent in general practice. In four cases there was a failure to explore a patient's beliefs and concerns about their problem: this also led to non-attendance at secondary care. Insufficient reassurance was given for two patients with self limiting problems (an infant with facial warts and a young child with obstructed tear duct): parental pressure to

Reason for referral	Referral appropriate	Referral avoidable
Specialist skills or procedure	54 (32)	7 (4)
Lack of knowledge	13 (7)	7 (4)
Lack of resources	12 (7)	32 (19)
Other perspective or view	31 (18)	12 (7)
Total	110 (64)	58 (34)

Evaluation of appropriateness of 168 referrals of patients to secondary care by a general practitioner. Values are numbers (percentages)

refer had been applied, but the problems had resolved before an appointment at outpatient department had been issued and the patients did not attend at the specialist clinics. A need for more knowledge was identified in seven cases, when failure either to know or at least to follow a recognised and readily available management plan led to avoidable referrals.

The need to acquire certain skills was identified in seven avoidable referrals. Three patients needed proctoscopy, and disposable proctoscopes should have been available in each examination room. Expertise in cleaning the auditory canal (two cases) and cryotherapy for warts (two cases) were also unavailable in the practice at the time of the study.

Discussion

Of the referrals studied, 34% were deemed to be avoidable in this singlehanded practice. Most of the avoidable referrals were caused by a lack of resources (32/58 (72%)). It should be noted, however, that 22 of these referrals were really only theoretically avoidable – for example, not having access to a community psychiatric nurse meant that the failure to refer within primary care was unavoidable. Nevertheless, theory could so easily be translated into practice provided there are real shifts in resources towards general practitioners.

Ten of the avoidable referrals were due to inadequate hospital information about earlier contacts with the patient (see box for examples), confirming the potentially high costs that can result from poor communication. It could be argued that the referring doctor should have spent more time requesting this information, but the reality is that in a busy practice it is not practical to spend time in pursuit of missing information when other priorities are pressing. It is quicker to write a referral letter, particularly if the doctor thinks that the referral may be necessary anyway.

Easy access to community psychiatric nurses would have improved access to information about secondary care in five cases, and in two others a community psychiatric nurse (if available) could have helped with a home based alcohol detoxification programme. Nursing support for palliative care may have reduced the likelihood of medical referral in five cases. Lack of direct access to day hospital (three referrals), general practitioner beds (two referrals), or professions allied to medicine (three referrals) also contributed to the avoidable referrals to specialists. Fundholding general practices would be expected to buy the above services, but confusion over responsibilities at the interface between generalists and specialists is also an issue. The trust between a general practitioner and a patient is easily damaged if specialists' plans for that patient bypass the general practitioner, and unnecessary referrals or admissions are easily precipitated by such lack of professional manners and etiquette.

Many of the 26 avoidable referrals that were due to limitations of knowledge, attitude, or skills could have been pre-empted by referrals within a group practice. A singlehanded doctor does not have this option, but it is widely practised in Canada, where family doctors often have specialist interests. General practitioners' time is, however, at a premium in the new NHS, so that changes in this area may be slow unless internal referral becomes recognised as part of normal practice and the calculations of the workforce in general practice are reviewed to allow for the rising pressure on British general practitioners since 1990.[7]

Our findings in a singlehanded practice may not be generalisable to others. However, a method that invokes an in depth review of the referral process is more likely to produce practical context specific suggestions for change than a population based methodology which searches for broader explanatory variables, targets, guidelines, rules or other generalisations that are not context sensitive. The next stage in the development of our method would be to apply it to a wider sample of practices. This would test our results and provide a basis for the definition of core skills for general practitioners.

Conclusion

Independent peer review is challenging for general practitioners because it provides an assessment of needs and raises organisation, resource and personal issues to address. This study also provided more evidence to justify transfer of local resources from secondary to primary care, and it confirmed the high cost of poor communication between secondary and primary care. There is some encouraging evidence of improved communication between 1991 and 1993,[8] but among both doctors and managers of hospitals there is still room for improvement. We conclude that general practitioners could reduce demands on specialists if the workforce in primary care was increased sufficiently to cope with demand, if there was easy access to intermediate care, if there was an improvement in communication between hospitals and general practices, and if the team resources available to general practitioners were enhanced and managed in house. We plan a larger study with similar methodology to test our conclusions on a more representative sample of general practitioners.

Examples of poor communication by hospitals

Case 1 – A 71-year-old man had been seen by a urology department because of outflow obstruction and recurrent urinary tract infections. He had received an intravenous pyelogram and was discharged in July, having been told that the result would be reviewed at the outpatient department in the near future. In October of the same year he contacted his general practitioner and queried the arrangements for follow up at the outpatient department. Although it was possible to obtain a verbal report of the intravenous pyelogram – 'A smallish right kidney' – this was not sufficient to allow the patient to be advised, and he was referred again to the urology department. Improved communication in terms of speed and content would have enabled this patient to have been managed in general practice.

Case 2 – A 25-year-old man was discharged from hospital after arthroscopy of the right shoulder. His general practitioner did not receive any information about the operation, and apparently no indication was given to the patient about future management or the suitability of returning to work. In view of this lack of information, the patient was referred back to the orthopaedic outpatient department.

Practice implications

- General practitioners' rates of referral vary widely, but relatively few studies have made objective attempts to assess how many referrals to hospitals might be avoided.

- In this study a general practitioner reviewed the appropriateness of 170 of his referrals with an independent assessor.

- A third of referrals were considered to be at least theoretically avoidable if adequate resources and direct access to intermediary care were available.

- Poor communication with hospitals about patients who had been discharged was another reason for avoidable referrals.

- Demand on secondary care could be reduced if workforce and resources in primary care were made sufficient to cope with demand and if communication between hospitals and general practitioners was improved.

1 Wilkin D. Patterns of referral: explaining variation in hospital referrals. In: Roland M, Coulter A, Eds. *Hospital referrals*. Oxford: Oxford University Press, 1992: 76-91.

2 Moore A T, Roland M O. How much variation in referral rates among general practitioners is due to chance? BMJ 1989; **298**: 5400-502.

3 Stott N C H. Help seeking behaviour. *In: Primary health care: bridging the gap between theory and practice*. Berlin: Springer Verlag, 1983: 43-51.

4 NHS Management Executive. What do we mean by appropriate health care? *Quality in Health Care* 1993; **2**: 117-23.

5 McWinney L R. *Textbook of family med-icine*. Oxford: Oxford University Press, 1989: 45-78.

6 Fertig A, Rowland M, King H, Moore T. Understanding variation in rates of referral among general practitioners: are inappropriate referrals important and would guidelines help reduce rates? BMJ 1993; **307**: 1467-70.

7 Stott N C H. The new general practitioner? Br. J. Gen. Pract. 1994; **44**: 2-3.

8 Pill R M, Smithers M, *Health services for residents of south Glamorgan: a report on the results of a survey of general practitioners*. Cardiff: University of Wales, College of Medicine 1993:20–1.

Evaluation of primary nursing in a nursing development unit

RESOURCE 3

Nursing Times, (Sept. 26, Vol. 91, No. 39, 1995)

Key words

Organisation of care, audit.

Abstract

This paper describes the method by which the staff team on a nursing development unit audited the way in which they organised the delivery of nursing care. Through the use of an established audit tool they were able to learn about their own practice as well as offering a critique of the tool.

Carolyn Mills, RGN, BSc, PGCEA, project leader/clinical nurse specialist, intensive care/nursing development unit, Chelsea and Westminster Hospital, London.

The three documents *The Patient's Charter, A Vision for the Future* and *A Strategy for Nursing* [1-3] advocate using primary nursing as an organisational approach to care, recognising its potential to enhance practice.

It cannot be stated categorically whether primary nursing is better than other ways of organising care, although some evidence suggests some improved outcomes. [4,5,6]

Primary nursing as an organisational approach to care has several identified benefits for patients, families, nurses and other members of the multidisciplinary team. Some of these are supported by research and some are drawn from the literature.

The value of primary nursing would appear to lie not in its approach but as a philosophy, enabling nurses to practise in ways that reflect what nursing means to them. [7] From this perspective the benefits to patients would result indirectly through greater autonomy, responsibility and subsequent job satisfaction for practising nurses. [8]

Truth Ward Nursing Development Unit (NDU) has been practising primary nursing for the past two years. Primary nursing matches the values and beliefs that the staff hold about nursing. Subjectively, primary nursing is positively evaluated by the nursing staff, who feel that they can get to know patients and families better. This facilitates increased quality of care and more satisfaction for nurses, patients and families.

We are continually striving to improve, develop and evaluate our practice. One of the identified responsibilities of NDUs is 'to open their work to critical evaluation, seeking formal evidence of the efficiency and effectiveness of their practice, and to assess the quality of their service as a means of monitoring progress as well as identifying new areas for development'. [9]

Our perception that we were practising primary nursing was subjective, the organisational approach to care never having been audited formally. We had also identified from our practice areas in the organisation of primary nursing that could be further developed to enhance our standard of care.

To help identify areas for improvement, and to validate or reject our previous subjective evaluation, we decided to audit the organisational approach to care on the ward.

Primary nursing is not easy to evaluate as much of the work involved is difficult to measure. We chose to use a validated audit tool to clarify, understand and measure primary nursing as our work method. The use of a validated audit tool decreased the potential for subjectivity, which can be a problem in evaluation, and assisted us by giving direction to our practice development. It also provided us with some baseline data, which we could use for a comparison with data collected in other areas and from which lessons could be learnt.

The audit tool

Care organisation needs to be audited in order to guide practice development. There are many tools available, but few are user-friendly, easy to understand and research-based. The 7E Nursing Development Unit at the John Radcliffe Hospital in Oxford had recently used and evaluated three care delivery audit tools. [10]

Having studied their report and critique, we decided to use one designed by Bowman, Webster and Thompson. [11] It seemed to offer a more sophisticated analysis of care organisation than the others and acknowledges the dynamic nature of our work. [10]

The tool is identified as a classification system for the clarification, understanding and measurement of nurses' work methods and was developed from an extensive review of the literature concerning various work methods. [11] The classification system was developed to distinguish between primary nursing, team nursing and task allocation. The authors assumed that each method of organising care facilitated different types of nurse-patient interaction, with primary nursing providing the greatest opportunity for interaction and task allocation the least. The strength of opportunity within the three categories was arbitrarily categorised as strong, moderate or weak (Table 1).

The work method assessment sheet has 13 components, of which 11 are scored based on interviews with nurses and two based on patients' views. The auditors allocated scores between one and four for each possible response: the higher the score, the greater the potential indicated for nurse-patient interaction.

The auditor would then allocate the score that most closely matched the interviewee's response. For example, if the response to question 7 was 'sister makes all the decisions' the auditor would judge the sister's role to be central and the score would be one with a weak opportunity for nurse-patient interaction (Table 1). However, if the response was 'sister supports us but does not interfere', the auditor would judge that the sister worked mainly in an advisory role and the score would be three (Table 1).

The resulting scores, therefore, reflect whether interactions were on an individual basis with a registered nurse (primary), with a small group (team) or with any nurse from the ward (task allocation).

Bowman et al. said the tool was 'crude and required refinement' and the auditors on 7E reiterated this and identified several specific areas for development.[10] We decided to use the audit tool as it was, while remaining aware of the criticisms raised. To refine it further would have required considerable time. We had already planned areas of development within our practice of primary nursing, and we wanted to audit our organisation of care before we implemented any changes. Undertaking the audit at this time provided us with baseline data that could be compared with data collected once planned changes had been established, allowing us to assess the effects of these changes.

	Primary			Team			Task		
	S	M	W	S	M	W	S	M	W
7 What is the sister's role in making decisions about nursing care?	3	2	2	2	1	1	1	1	1
a) central									✓
b) advisory									
c) a mixture	✓								
8 Who generally discusses the patient's nursing care with the medical and paramedical staff?	3	2	2	2	1	1	1	1	1
a) the ward sister/charge nurse									
b) a named registered nurse all of the time									
c) any nurse available									
12. (To be asked of patient.) How often is the patient involved in decisions related to nursing care?	4	4	3	3	3	2	2	2	1
a) nearly always									
b) frequently									
c) rarely									
d) never									

Key: S = strong, M = moderate, W = weak

Table 1: A work method assessment sheet with examples of two scores

Box 1. Identified areas for development

- To look at roles of associate and primary nurses, and how these fit in with the wider organisational structure

- Specific areas for development within the role of the primary nurse related to care planning, patterns of responsibility, authority, accountability, autonomy and advocacy

- To look at who is able to be a primary nurse, related to the perceived potential for devaluing associate nurses

- To look at ways of ensuring that nursing is the main focus in patient assessments and in care planning

- To look at ways of improving multidisciplinary care planning

- To look at ways of increasing the patients' awareness of primary nursing, what it is and how this will affect them during their admission

- To improve primary job satisfaction for nurses, associate nurses and other group members.

The tool seemed adequate for our purposes of providing some baseline data to guide our practice development. In the discussion of our evaluation we have noted the points raised in the evaluation in Oxford and have tried to clarify these areas for the purposes of our interpretation of the audit.

To increase the validity of results, and the reliability of the tool, two independent auditors carried out the audit. Anecdotal evidence was collected to substantiate the auditor's judgement. Consent was sought from the patients involved and the process explained to them before they were asked if they would participate.

Results

A pilot audit undertaken for the purpose of familiarisation (that did not examine care plans and did not involve patients) obtained a score of 37, indicating weak to moderate primary nursing. The actual score obtained in the audit on Truth Ward was 33. This indicated that the work method on Truth Ward was strong to moderate team nursing. It highlighted the difference between the auditors' perception of how the nurses' work was organised and how it actually was.

This was a disappointing result, but it needs to be placed in context. At the time that the audit was carried out, the structure of the ward team had been altered in response to staff shortage. This increased each primary nurse's patient case load from seven to 10 or 11 patients. The maximum

recommended number of patients for one primary nurse to look after effectively is six.[11]

At the time of the audit, the hospital was undergoing a period of considerable organisational and structural change. There were also some new staff who may not have developed an understanding of the theory, practice and organisation of primary nursing.

The tool was easy to use, and the nurses carrying out the audit were helped by the previous critique of the model.[10]

Conclusions

The areas for development identified by the audit are outlined in Box 1. Action plans were drawn up to look at specific ways of achieving our aims in relation to the developmental areas identified in the audit. Further evaluation was planned (Box 2).

Despite its limitations, the tool offered us a way of classifying, clarifying, understanding and measuring the nurses' organisation of care. The information obtained allowed us to identify areas of our practice in the organisation of care that we did well, and those areas that could benefit from development. The audit also highlights the importance of evaluating established practices that could be forgotten after new developments.

Established practice developments need to be evaluated if they are to continue to develop, to ensure they remain effective and contribute to the overall standard of care we can offer our patients.

> ## Box 2. Further evaluation
>
> - Ongoing evaluation through clinical supervision of all staff
>
> - Evaluation in six months. This will be done using the same audit tool and will be carried out by the same two auditors, to evaluate the effectiveness of the development strategies instigated following the previous audit.

References

1 Department of Health. *The Patient's Charter*. London: HMSO, 1991.

2 Department of Health. *A Vision for the Future*. London: HMSO, 1993.

3 Department of Health. *A Strategy for Nursing*. London: HMSO, 1989.

4 Culpepper, R., Sinclair, V., Betz, M. The effects of primary nursing on nursing quality assurance. *Journal of Nursing Administration* 1986; 16: 11, 24-31.

5 Manley, K. *Primary nursing in critical care*. London: Scutari, 1989.

6 Giovanetti, P., Evaluation of primary nursing. In: *Annual Review of Nursing Research* 1986; 4: 127-51.

7 Ersser, S., Tutton, E. (eds.) *Primary Nursing in Perspective*. Harrow: Scutari, 1991.

8 Vaughan, B. The pursuit of excellence. *Nursing Times* 1992; 88: 31, 26-29.

9 Adair, L., Murray, L. Organisation of nursing care project. In: Bowman, G., Thompson, D. (eds.) A Classification System for Nurses' Work Methods: *The Bowman Classification*. Oxford: National Institute for Nursing, 1995.

10 Bowman, G., Webster, R., Thompson, D. The development of a classification system for nurses' work methods. *International Journal of Nursing Studies* 1991; 28: 2, 175-187.

11 Hegyvary, S. *The Change to Primary Nursing*. St Louis, Missouri: Mosby, 1982.

RESOURCE 4

Evaluation and the Health Profession, (Vol.16, No.4, Dec. 1993)

Using qualitative methods to evaluate health service delivery in three rural Colorado communities

Qualitative and quantitative methods can be used simultaneously for hypothesis generation and testing. A pilot study was conducted in 1991 in three rural Colorado communities to clarify health service delivery problems related to cancer. The analysis focused on the perceptions of three types of respondents in each community related to whether cancer was a major problem, whether health services were adequate in their community and what perceived solutions could be implemented. Respondents included community influentials, health care providers and cancer patients or family members. Semi-structured phone interviews were used to collect perceptions of these community members. Transcripts from the three communities were combined, coded and tallied. Several distinct themes emerged from the analysis. These included: cancer was a major problem; public and provider education was needed; community systems and support to identify and solve health problems were lacking; medical networking needed to be expanded; transportation was a problem for remote communities; inability to pay for services was a problem for rural communities. Most respondents identified the problems as relevant to other chronic and acute diseases as well as cancer. This method identified the critical problems for the majority of the people without losing sight of the outlier responses.

Authors' note

Thanks go to our team of consultants, who

assisted in making this inquiry rich with detail and useful for understanding rural health care ecology: Jeanne Nicholson, Gilpin County Nursing Service; Marguerite Salazar, Valleywide Health Center; Larry Dunn, Cooperative Extension Service Rural Development; Susan Hill, Colorado Action for Healthy People; Lindy Nelson, Colorado Department of Health; Richard Bakemeier, University of Colorado Cancer Center; Rich Call, Area Health Education Centers. Thanks go also to Stuart Cohen and Don Iverson for assistance in seminal ideas and development of this project; John Berg for his contribution in the quantitative analysis of CCCR data; Deborah Nelson, Karin Hohman and Karen Brekke for assistance in interview development and execution; and to the many others who have encouraged our team and contributed to this effort.

Quantitative analysis is often employed in health care research to provide a statistical comparison of two or more treatment modalities, groups of patients or sets of interventions. On the other hand, qualitative research is more frequently used in health education or intervention development as a way to measure whether an intervention was implemented as planned, to assess the target audience's perception of an intervention or to provide insights into an audience's beliefs or knowledge about an issue (Eriksson, 1988). Qualitative analysis is usually performed to generate hypotheses or to develop programs, whereas quantitative analysis is most often used for actual hypothesis testing (Buchanan, 1992).

This article reviews the traditional uses of qualitative and quantitative evaluation and describes the application of qualitative analysis for hypothesis generation and inquiry. We conducted a study using qualitative techniques to help clarify health service delivery problems in selected rural areas in Colorado. The object was to determine whether generic problems existed and to assess the perception of solutions to these problems from the communities that experienced them.

Qualitative and quantitative evaluation

Qualitative and quantitative methods differ in their traditional uses, objectives, methods and modes of analysis (DeVries, Weijts, Dijkstra, & Kok, 1992). Quantitative methods are based upon the empirical paradigm of the physical sciences (DeVries et al., 1992; Steckler, McLeroy, Goodman, Bird, & McCormick, 1992), which predicts relationships between variables. Qualitative analysis is based upon the anthropological sciences' paradigm of observation (DeVries et al., 1992, Steckler et al., 1992), in which data are analysed through the language of communication and insight of perceptions,

reactions and consequences of behavior. Because of these differences, qualitative analysis is seldom used alone. It is viewed as a subjective, inductive process of discovery as compared to the reliable, deductive method of quantitative analysis preferred by the majority of the scientific community and by funding agencies in particular (Steckler et al., 1992). However, mainstream quantitative methods provide limited information about human intentions and thought processes that underlie overt behaviors.

Because several tasks are important for a complete understanding of a program or problem (i.e. monitoring, impact assessment and causal explanation; Eriksson, 1988), qualitative and quantitative analysis can and should be used together. Steckler et al. (1992) outline several different ways this can be achieved. Qualitative or quantitative methods can be used to explain the results obtained from the other (e.g. using quantitative survey results to identify whether an opinion obtained from a qualitative interview is representative, or using a focus group to provide details about the particular target groups for which a barrier has been identified in a survey). Another way to combine the methodologies is to use qualitative methods to develop more empirical quantitative measures (e.g. ethnographic interviewing to prepare for questionnaire construction; Bauman & Adair, 1992). Lastly, the two methods can be used equally to cross-validate findings, thereby strengthening confidence in the results and conclusions. This method, called triangulation, is common (Patton, 1990), but it is most often used with multiple methods that are primarily qualitative or quantitative. Recommendations for increasing confidence in qualitative assessment include studying the population for a longer period of time to reduce the likelihood of distorted data (prolonged engagement) and gathering information from several different sources (triangulation) to increase the representativeness of the sample.

Combining qualitative and quantitative methods: an example

Prior to development of a community-based cancer control intervention, real and perceived health care problems in rural areas in Colorado needed to be defined. Residents of rural Colorado counties are similar to those elsewhere in rural America in terms of age, employment and health status. Specifically, rural residents are older, less educated and more often poor, unemployed or underemployed (Cordes, 1989), than their urban counterparts, and a greater proportion of rural Americans are in fair or poor health (15% vs. 10.9%) or suffer from chronic or serious illness (23.4% vs. 18.7%) (Robert Wood Johnson Foundation, 1987). These conditions increase an individual's susceptibility to disease (Breslow, 1990; Kovar, 1982). Geographic and resource isolation, coupled with political and social disadvantages, contribute to health service resource shortages in rural areas as well (General Accounting Office, 1978; Moscovice, 1989; Pomeranz & Rosenberg, 1985/1986; Sharp, Halpert, & Breytspraak, 1988; Van Hook, 1988; Williams, Schwartz, Newhouse, & Bennett, 1983). However, according to the 1988 Colorado Central Cancer Registry (CCCR) (report by J. Berg, personal communication, 1991), the stage of diagnosis of preventable cancers (i.e. bowel, cervix, breast, prostate), which is related to access to health care services, was not significantly different for all rural counties combined (as defined by nonmetropolitan statistical areas) than for all urban counties (total metropolitan statistical areas). For bowel cancers, 29% of staged cancers were localised in both rural and urban areas. Comparing stage of diagnosis of cancer by geography, 5.5 times as many in situ cervical cancers as invasive cancers were found in the rural areas, as compared to 3.3 times as many in situ as invasive for the combined rural and urban areas, suggesting adequacy of screening exams in rural areas. For breast cancer, 63% of statewide and 64% of rural cancers were insitu or localised. Nor were differences found between rural and urban counties for diagnosis to treatment time (D-T time) of preventable cancers. Observed/expected ratios were constructed for all patients waiting more than a month for treatment. The range of D-T ratios for urban areas was 0.6-1.7 (unweighted mean for 10 SMSA counties was 0.7), whereas the mean D-T ratio for rural areas was 1.2. Given these quantitative study results, we could conclude that access to care in rural Colorado areas was similar to that in more urban parts of the state because early stage of diagnosis and time to treatment were similar.

An assumption was made that the real problems in rural Colorado communities were not reflected in the data from the CCCR. A broader view of the perception of cancer-related and health service delivery problems that exist in these communities was sought and was the basis for this qualitative assessment. The opinions of residents imbedded in the economic and social contexts in which they live could lead to a very different inference than derived from the CCCR data or from a quantitative assessment of hospital bed days or survival figures. Although universal themes might result from a qualitative assessment of the opinions and ideas in this population, divergent and unique ideas could also emerge and lead to creative solutions to the problems identified.

A pilot study was undertaken in the spring of 1991 to evaluate the perceptions of a wide range of rural health care users and providers regarding cancer-related problems and solutions in three different rural communities in Colorado. The analysis focused on three research questions:

1 Is cancer a major problem in the community?
2 What are the perceptions of health service delivery problems in the community and are they related to cancer?
3 What solutions to these perceived health service delivery problems are currently or potentially being implemented in the community?

Methods

Community selection

Information about Colorado's 63 counties was collected to identify a variety of population characteristics, including: size and age of population, ethnicity/race, population density, provision of local health care services and infant mortality rate. Counties were classified as adjacent rural (rural yet sustain services that are tertiary in nature), countryside rural (communities with fewer than 2,500 residents or counties with fewer than 100,000 residents and not adjacent to metropolitan areas) and frontier rural (counties with fewer than six people per square mile) (Fickenscher, 1990). Using these definitions and an array of variables from sources such as the U.S. Census Bureau, Area Resource File, Colorado County Health Profiles and Directory of Colorado Health Facilities, three communities were chosen to represent the diversity of rural areas in the state. These communities were Greeley in Weld County (adjacent), Eagle in Eagle County (countryside) and San Louis in Costilla County (frontier). Table 1 indicates the range of variables used in selecting communities.

Characteristic	Costilla	Eagle	Weld
Rural classification	Frontier	Countryside	Adjacent
Percent Hispanic	77.5	9.3	17.0
Percent urban	0.0	0.0	57.3
People/square mile	2.7	11.7	35.0
People/primary care doctors	3345	1742	2859
Number hospitals	0	1	2
Percent population in poverty	36.1	9.4	14.1
Percent population >65 yrs	13.8	3.0	8.8
5 yr infant mortality rate	6.8	7.3	9.2
Health manpower shortage area	Yes	No	Yes

Note: Data based on the following years: % Hispanic (1980); % urban (1980); People/square mile (1987); People/primary-care doctor (1986); Number hospitals (1990); % population in poverty (1979); % population >65 (1980); 5 yr infant mortality rate (1979-1983); HMSA (1987).

Table 1: Community characteristics of three rural communities

Respondent selection

In each community, study participants included:

1 community influentials (e.g. school teachers, librarians, directors of community agencies, business leaders)
2 health care providers (i.e. physicians, nurses, public health personnel)
3 patients or family members of patients who had a cancer experience (i.e. screening, diagnosis, treatment and follow-up, rehabilitation or hospice).

Contacts in the State Health Department, Area Health Education Center, the Colorado Community Health Network and the Cooperative Extension Service helped identify a primary contact person in each of the three communities. These individuals exhibited global community awareness and an ability to point out other key informants in the community. During a period of 6 weeks (prolonged engagement), these community contacts referred us to key influentials, health care providers and patients/family members (triangulation). In each community 8 to 14 individuals, distributed among the three types of respondents, were contacted. These participants were queried about their perceptions of problems related to health service delivery for cancer and other health issues and were prompted to suggest solutions for these problems.

Method selection and development

Semistructured in-depth telephone interviews were chosen as the methods of inquiry because of the potential for richness of data collected while still focusing on specific issues through a structured format. The research team developed four interviews to evaluate the experiences and perceptions of the three types of respondents. Each interview format was pretested with appropriate respondent samples and revised accordingly.

Performing the interviews

All telephone interviews were conducted by trained research staff; interviews were taped and transcribed. Patient interviews focused on the ease of entry into the health care system, use of local and distant medical services, systems of referral, adequacy of services, transportation and financial barriers, quality of care and follow-up care. Questions included, 'Were you able to get all the medical services you needed? Where did you go to get the medical services you needed?' Interviewers encouraged patients to offer suggestions for improvement in cancer screening, diagnosis, treatment and/or rehabilitative care. Patients were also asked to specify the single largest health care problem in their community.

For the health care providers, two interviews were used: one for clinicians and another for public health-orientated personnel. For the clinician interviews, scenarios that described potential cancer-related issues in rural health care elicited two responses. Following is one of three scenarios used:

Mrs Smith, a 42-year-old woman whom you have never seen before other than when she brought one of her children in for an earache a few months ago, presents with a painless mass in her left breast. She is recently divorced and currently has no health insurance. Other than her children, there are no immediate family members in the commu-

nity. Mammography is obtained and reveals a suspicious area in the breast highly suggestive of malignancy.

Clinicians were asked to describe the current approach in using existing health care systems for each scenario, pointing out gaps in those services/ systems. They then were prompted to provide solutions that might improve the system. Additional questions elicited their perception of the largest health and cancer-related problems in the community and solutions for affecting both.

Health care providers who were public health orientated responded to both the clinical scenario and a scenario about communitywide issues. For the clinical scenario, they were asked to consider access, referrals, transportation, cost and other barriers in recommending treatment and to provide solutions to the problems which they identified. The community scenario was as follows:

Think about an important cancer-related health problem in your community. This could be something like alcohol abuse, lack of health care services or public misinformation about cancer. Briefly describe that problem. How do you use existing community systems and resources to deal with that problem? What changes in your community's systems or resources do you believe would improve the cancer-related issue you describe?

As with the clinical interview, additional questions were asked about the largest health and cancer-related problems in the community and solutions for both.

For the community influential interview, the same questions about community-wide issues were used. Each participant was asked to respond as a recognised leader with community-wide perspective in considering what changes in the community's current systems or resources might enhance health services. To provide community context, influentials were queried about other health-related programs that had been implemented locally and asked how to improve similar programs in the future. Participants assessed the importance of cancer as a health issue in their community and their perceptions of the major health care problems locally.

Analysis

Transcripts from the three communities were combined to identify the range of issues faced by the three types of rural communities. These were divided into the three categories of interview: key influential, health care provider and cancer patient/family member. Transcripts were identified by code to assure anonymity. Two independent staff performed a blinded review of each transcript and coded sentences (Patton, 1980) that answered one of the three research questions: cancer as a major problem, problems related to cancer and solutions to cancer problems. These sentences were then classified as being a cancer problem only or as a problem related to health issues other than cancer. For each transcript, the two staff members reached a consensus about the category in which each sentence belonged. After all information in each transcript had been coded, all transcripts in each interview category (i.e. influential, provider, patient/family) were then collected and tallied. All information common to at least two separate transcripts was used for the final reporting.

Results

Tables 2 and 3 indicate problems and solutions identified during the interviews. A + indicates that two or more transcripts identified the item as a problem or a solution for either cancer-related health issues or for other health-related issues.

Universal themes

Distinct themes emerged from the analysis. Table 4 contains relevant quotes from the transcripts for the problems identified by individuals in the survey.

Cancer is a major problem. Providers, patients and community influentials identified cancer as a significant health care issue in their community.

Public and provider education is needed. Providers and influentials felt that community-wide education for increased awareness of cancer-related issues and services available would promote increased use of those services, alleviate fear and promote service expansion.

Community systems/support to identify and solve health problems are lacking. Providers primarily identified the need for organisation of local and nonlocal resources and coordination of efforts to provide continuity of care.

Medical networking needs to be expanded. Providers felt that networking with local and nonlocal health organisations would maximise the use of limited resources.

Lack of transportation is a hardship for remote communities. Providers described the inability of some patient populations to obtain care due to distance to services.

Inability to pay for services is a problem for most rural populations. Providers, patients and influentials all noted the difficulties in providing health services due to lack of insurance, financing and unstable economies that cannot provide services for all underserved populations. Lack of financing also contributes to health provider shortages in rural areas.

Although most of the specific questions were framed within a context of health service delivery for cancer care, most community respondents identified the problems as relevant to other chronic and acute disease treatment and prevention issues in their communities.

Issues	Cancer-Related			Other Health-Related		
	Provider	Patient	Influential	Provider	Patient	Influential
Cancer a major problem	+	+	+			
Finance/cost/insurance	+		+	+	+	+
Public education	+		+	+		
Inadequate local services	+	+	+	+	+	+
Transportation	+				+	
Medical networking	+			+		
Community systems	+		+			
Support services				+		+
Health beliefs/fears			+			
Primary prevention		+	+			
Secondary prevention		+	+			
Substance abuse						+
Special populations				+		
Chronic disease				+		+
Child/teen health						+

Table 2: Problem identification

Issues	Cancer-Related			Other Health-Related		
	Provider	Patient	Influential	Provider	Patient	Influential
Public education	+		+	+		+
Professional education/ medical networking	+		+	+		+
Enhanced health services	+	+	+	+	+	+
Enhanced support services	+		+	+		+
Community organisation			+	+		+
Cost/finance/insurance	+	+	+	+		
Local subsidy for services	+					
Transportation	+			+		+

Table 3: Solution identification

Physicians/health care providers:

Regional facilities only accept paying patients or close down.

The remoteness of the community creates a lack of services.

Physician shortage exists because of low salaries, large workloads and difficult patients.

We don't have training or equipment to do high-tech care.

Community influentials:

People are on waiting lists for services for several months.

There are not enough professionals or volunteers here.

There is inadequate provider knowledge about specialised services.

Patients/family members:

A time or two we have had no doctor here.

We have a doctor here now but his patients have no money and I hear he's going to leave.

We need treatment locally.

I was on a waiting list for 3 weeks before the mammography van got here.

Table 4: Selected perceptions about local health services by interview respondents

Discussion

This qualitative analysis of three rural communities (adjacent, countryside, frontier) in Colorado was conducted to evaluate the perceptions of problems with health care systems related to cancer. The pilot occurred during a 3-month period in 1991. The analysis suggests that cancer is a significant problem in these three rural communities in Colorado. Issues related to inadequacy of services for cancer and other health care included: financial resources with which to obtain cancer-related care, cancer and health care public education, local health services, transportation to seek care, networking among health care providers (locally and nonlocally), community systems to identify and solve problems and community support services. Respondents also identified barriers related to health beliefs or fears, and problems related to the presence of special populations non acculturated to the existing medical care system. Participants suggested such solutions as public education, enhanced local health care services, improved community support services, community organisation activities, health professional education and networking, affordable screening, increased financial resources for health care and expanded transportation.

The largest problems for the majority of people were identified as being the most important without losing sight of the outlier responses nor the social context within which the reports were made. This is similar to a quantitative approach but without washing out the rich detail found in opposing viewpoints. A qualitative approach also provided

this research team with the impetus to design an intervention flexible enough to affect health service delivery in a variety of communities where the perception of the problems may differ but the result of the service gap is similar.

This qualitative assessment does not provide conclusive evidence about the major public health problems related to health service delivery in rural Colorado. Although an attempt was made to gather data from a diverse set of communities (n = 3) and a variety of individuals within those communities (n = 31), the sample size was small and the key influential individuals were those who had a certain status within the community and could be identified by others as having an opinion. In addition, the three communities chosen are mostly dependent upon farming, ranching and tourism, whereas other major industries in Colorado include mining, service, education, gambling and manufacturing, thus providing an economic and political context for the issues that were defined.

As noted, qualitative analysis attempts to gain broader insights into the human perceptions and behaviors through observation and discussion, rather than through random sampling. This analysis provided several benefits over a traditional quantitative inquiry into the problems and solutions in health service delivery related to cancer in rural Colorado. First, respondents were able to identify and prioritise problems in their communities independent of the perceptions of other community members. This fostered a non-biased response, as each interview was conducted in a non-suggestive format without input from others. Our study also analysed perceptions of the systems by those who provided the care, those who experienced the care and those who had a sense of the larger community care needs. This provided an insider's view from multiple vantage points. Moreover, this method encouraged the generation of creative ideas for solutions to the problems that each individual perceived as important. Thus, these varied participants' ideas spanned a broader range of problems than would be provided by a consensus approach to problem and solution identification. Lastly, a flexible intervention based upon these community perceptions was developed for testing in other similar rural Colorado communities.

Conclusions

Qualitative analysis provided a relatively efficient, low-cost method of assessing the health service issues in a triad of rural Colorado communities. In combination with quantitative information, this method provides considerable context for understanding the perceptions as well as the realities of rural Colorado. This method may also have promise for understanding rural health service issues beyond cancer.

References

Bauman, L.J. & Adair, E.G. (1992). The use of ethnographic interviewing to inform questionnaire construction. *Health Education Quarterly*, 19(1), 9-23.

Breslow, L., (1990). The future of public health: Prospects in the US for the 90s. *Annual Review of Public Health*, 11, 1-28.

Buchanan, D. R. (1992).An uneasy alliance: Combining qualitative and quantitative research methods. *Health Education Quarterly*, 19(1), 117-135.

Cordes, S.M. (1989). The changing rural environment and the relationship between health services and rural development. *Health Services Research*, 23(6), 757-784.

DeVries, H., Weijts, W., Dijkstra, M. & Kok, G. (1992). The utilisation of qualitative and quantitative data for health education program planning, implementation and evaluation: A spiral approach. *Health Education Quarterly*, 19(1), 101-115.

Eriksson, C.G. (1988). Focus groups and other methods for increased effectiveness of community intervention: A review. *Scandinavian Journal of Primary Health Care Supplement*, 1, 73-80.

Fickenscher, K. (1990). *Research on primary care and rural health: Opportunities and challenges.* Paper presented at the meeting of the Agency for Health Care Policy and Research, Colorado Springs, CO.

General Accounting Office. (1978). *Progress and problems in improving the availability of primary care providers in underserved areas.* Washington, DC: Author.

Kovar, M.G. (1982). Health status of US children and use of medical care. *Public Health Report*, 97(1), 3-5.

Moscovice, I. (1989). Strategies for promoting a viable rural health care system. *Journal of Rural Health*, 5(3), 216-230.

Patton, M.Q. (1980). *Qualitative evaluation methods.* Beverly Hills, CA: Sage.

Patton, M.Q. (1990). *Qualitative evaluation and research methods.* Newbury Park, CA: Sage.

Pomeranz, W. & Rosenberg, S. (1985/1986). Developing home health services in rural communities – An innovative solution to a thorny problem. *Home Health Services Quarterly*, 6(4), 5-10.

Robert Wood Johnson Foundation. (1987). *Access to health care in the United States: Results of a 1986 survey*, No.2. Princeton, NJ: Author.

Sharp, T.S., Halpert, B.P. & Breytspraak, L.M. (1988). Impact of Medicare's prospective payment system and the farm crisis on the health care of the elderly: A case study. *Journal of Rural Health*, 4(3), 45-56.

Steckler, A., McLeroy, K.R., Goodman, R.M., Bird, S.T. & McCormick, L. (1992). Toward integrating qualitative and quantitative methods: An introduction. *Health Education Quarterly*, 19(1), 1-8.

Van Hook, R.T. (1988). The challenge of rural health. *Business Health*, 6(2), 406.

Williams, A.P., Schwartz, W.B., Newhouse, J.P. & Bennett, B.W. (1983). How many miles to the doctor? *New England Journal of Medicine.* 309(16), 958-963.

RESOURCE 5

David Hailey. From
Daly, Willis &
MacDonald (eds)
*Researching Health Care:
designs, dilemmas,
disciplines. Routledge,
1992.*

The perspective of the policymaker on health care research and evaluation

This contribution is given from the perspective of the Australian Institute of Health, an agency which informs the policy process rather than formulating policy itself. Probably the best customers for the various evaluation and statistical development activities at the Institute are policy areas in government. Policy areas outside health authorities are also important but government agencies tend to dominate consideration because of their closeness to decisions that will eventually affect the funding of health care programs.

Although most of this publication is concerned with the details of evaluation methodology, it is worth setting part of the scene by commenting on the nature of the policy process and the climate in which those responsible for formulating policy have to operate. After all, much of the purpose for attempting the difficult and costly process of health care evaluation is to influence the decisions taken by governments and others. To succeed in this dubious task it is as well to have some appreciation of the nature of the target.

Characteristics of policy areas

Pressing concerns for the policy makers in health authorities include the immediate directions of the Minister and the wishes of the government of the day, limited budgets for an apparently ever-expanding set of responsibilities, the relationship to coordinating departments and the short time scale in which decisions often have to be taken and results judged. Policy areas will often be under pressure to come up with something definite relatively quickly.

Other realities are that the policy maker will have to take on board a very broad perspective of the requirements in the health portfolio (considerably beyond the range envisaged by the typical researcher), and will need to respond to pressures, not only from the political arena, but also from professional groups. Typically, providers will be seeking access to government funds while health authorities will be defending their budgets.

Resulting action after a policy decision is taken may be difficult to reverse or adjust – for example, alteration to levels of reimbursement may be cumbersome to achieve.

Another characteristic seems to be a relatively rapid turnover of policy staff, perhaps associated with an increasing trend towards use of generalists. There may be capacity only for limited review and analysis and while control of health care programs may be significant there are limitations as to what can be achieved by a health authority. These features contribute to the caution shown in some policy making areas.

In recent years, cost containment has been a dominant theme, often at the expense of any major consideration of benefit from provision of health care programs. Frequently the constraints on the policy maker are such that a new initiative may be acceptable only if some alternative program can be reduced or given up. While policy makers may need to respond quickly they may also, in the interests of budgets or other government commitments, need to delay introduction of new health programs. There can be an interesting tension between the need for immediate advice and a bureaucratic preference for delay.

The policy maker will need to consider if the new health initiative will replace old methods or supplement them, or if it will have a significant effect on infrastructure. If so, will it be the responsibility of the area serviced by the health authority or can it be passed over to another level of government or to health insurance funds? In Australia, the split in responsibilities between Commonwealth and states adds to the complexity.

Evaluation and the policy process

Evaluation may often be seen by the policy maker as something of a wild card. Potentially, evaluation can help by providing data that can contribute to better-informed decision-making. Difficulties are that the evaluation data may not be easily assimilated into policy decisions, and in some cases may be regarded as embarrassing if they point to a need for significant change.

Evaluation is only one input to the policy making process. There are dangers for those who assess health care if it is not appreciated that the most elegant and detailed analysis may have no impact on the policy process and any subsequent action by government if the timing is wrong, the results are not presented in a way that is intelligible to policy makers or the recommendations are unrealistic in political terms.

The recent experience in Australia of introduction of Magnetic Resonance Imaging (MRI) services provides an illustration. Future policy on this expensive technology will be informed by the results of the Australian assessment program and by relevant data from overseas, but other impacts on the policy process will include pressures from coordinating departments, states, professional bodies, consumer organisations, manufacturing industry and various vested interest groups.

At present we are dealing with perhaps the fourth generation of persons in the relevant policy area since the MRI program started. Such turnover does not help in establishing some sort of understanding of the methods, strengths and constraints of evaluation.

I have noted elsewhere (Hailey, 1985) that in a climate where governments want results of assessments quickly, perhaps within 12 months and in appropriately brief form, it is difficult to encourage an appreciation of the need for detailed evaluation. The 'quick and nasty' approach can easily become the norm and carry greater weight with the policy maker than more detailed studies. Excellent proposals for evaluations will not necessarily attract support, and clinical studies of several years' duration do not sit casily with the imperatives implicit in the policy making process.

Some attitudes to evaluation

Comments made at the recent evaluation meeting organised by the Public Health Association (PHA) and the National Health and Medical Research Council (NHMRC) (PHA, 1989) provide some interesting insights into the perspectives of policy makers, though some of the views expressed may not be very comforting for researchers or evaluators.

The point was made that policy making in the health area has a relationship to the political process, which will include party politics. It is also closely related to power plays within the bureaucracy or involving it. It was suggested that one view of evaluation is that it helps the health authority to push away the problem – this is the idea of deferring the evil day when hard decisions might need to be made about support of a particular health care program. NHMRC was not seen as very relevant to the short term needs of the Commonwealth Department of Community Services and Health.

Consultants were seen as useful, as being able to generate quick opinions which departmental officers could choose to use or not,

as required – with no one else involved. (A counter view expressed was that often too little briefing and definition of tasks were provided to consultants and that insufficient funds were made available to them.) Perhaps more worrying, lack of control of evaluators was seen as a concern.

With these sort of attitudes, it may be difficult for researchers to judge the success of their work in terms of the health authority's view. From the policy maker's perspective, success through evaluation was seen in terms of providing new information, informing the policy process (including synthesis of available data), confirming the position previously adopted, and perhaps to bury a particular topic so that it could be filed and forgotten. It is very easy for government to file and forget things, and the view that the 'government knows' if the material is on file somewhere is not particularly helpful. The fact that the health authorities hold data does not mean that such information is necessarily relevant to the current decision-making process.

It was emphasised again at the PHA meeting that although research and evaluation can give useful input, policy formulation is a much broader process including, for example, relationships between the Commonwealth and state governments. I believe that, while this is true, at times there may be a tendency for policy areas to shelter behind this rationale to an unreasonable extent.

Need for communication and mutual education

Overall there seems to be a communication problem – a lack of contact between the policy areas and evaluators and, in turn, sometimes between the evaluation areas and professional groups. The policy area in a health authority to some extent has to be regarded by the evaluator as a 'black box', given the various additional inputs to the policy process both from within and outside departments. The concern of evaluators must be that the 'black box' does not develop into a black hole with data from research going in, but no relevant feedback being provided.

At the PHA meeting, Professor Gavin Mooney mentioned some of the barriers to evaluation influencing choice, if such choice exists. These include the management decision environment touched on already, the aloofness of professionals – Mooney talked in terms of the medical profession, but aloofness and reluctance to communicate with other disciplines are not peculiar to that group – the fact that health care is a highly political football, a suspicion of economists (and other evaluators) and a lack of advocacy.

The dilemma between desire for rapid input and the realities of lengthy evaluation periods emerges in all areas of health care, but is perhaps particularly apparent with the current interest in preventative measures and health promotion activities. Often the evaluation problems in these areas will be related to the need for long term protocols, countered by the wish of policy makers and governments to see a return on expenditure.

As noted by Penny Hawe, there are a series of problems in evaluating program effectiveness, including premature evaluation – looking for program effects before the program is functioning properly – evaluation without sufficient resources and results being ignored (Hawe, 1989). She also points out that process evaluation, impact evaluation and outcome evaluation have to be done in sequence to make sense. I see this providing a problem. There may be impatience on the part of policy areas with the process side of evaluation – that is, the necessary assurance that the program is working correctly before seeking measures of impact and outcome.

The needs of policy areas may include clear, realistic recommendations, a description of a health program from more than one aspect (considering perspectives other than those of its proponents) and overall appraisal of costs and benefits. There is still a problem for policy areas in considering benefits from health care programs. First, benefits are less easy to quantify than costs; second, they may have less impact on immediate policy pressures; and third, they may not be reflected in the budgets of those that pay for the programs. Finally, they may take a long time to emerge. There is also the familiar problem of the moving target, especially with some of the recent technologies and uncertainties regarding measurement of cost utilities.

Is all this a counsel for despair? I do not think so. There seems to me to be far greater acceptance of the need for evaluation of health care than was the case a few years ago. Some additional resources for evaluation are starting to emerge from governments. There is some appreciation that the assessment process can help and may be necessary for effective operation of health care programs.

Some of the more negative views of evaluation that seem common in policy areas may in the longer term be self-defeating, running the risk of leading to inefficient or unworkable health care programs. It seems to me that evaluation has to make data and analysis explicit, being itself open to challenge and subject to change.

I would see a need for evaluators to continue their efforts to communicate with policy areas, to describe health care programs clearly so that they are comprehensible to the policy advisers, and to provide analysis in intelligible terms on a short enough time scale. There is a major need for methods that are quick enough to inform the decision-making process adequately, in addition to longer term research.

In turn, policy areas need to develop approaches to be able to take on board results of longer term studies. What we need is evaluation which is better able to deal with the concerns and realities of the policy process and establish the essential place of assessment in consideration of health care.

References

Hailey, D.M., 1985, 'Health care technology assessment', in National Health and Medical Research Council (NHMRC), *Resources for Health Care Evaluation*, Canberra: NHMRC, 112-28.

Hawe, P., 1989, 'The last thing you should look at is cost effectiveness', in PHA, *National Health Care Evaluation Workshop*, Canberra: PHA.

Public Health Association of Australia (PHA), 1989, *National Health Care Evaluation Workshop*, Canberra: PHA.

REFERENCES

ABBOTT, P. and SAPSFORD, R. (1992) *Research into Practice: A reader for nurses and the caring professions*, Open University Press.

BARROWCLOUGH, C. and TARRIER, N. (1987) Assessing the functional value of relatives' knowledge about schizophrenia. *British Journal of Psychiatry*, **151**.

BARROWCLOUGH, C. and TARRIER, N. (1992) *Families of Schizophrenic Patients*, Chapman and Hall.

BRADSHAW, T. and EVERITT, J. (1995) 'Providing support for families', *Nursing Times*, Vol. **91**. No. 32.

CHEN, H. T. and ROSSI, P.H. (1983) 'Evaluating with sense: The theory-driven approach', *Evaluation Review*, **7**.

CLARK, E. (1987) *Research Awareness Module 5*, Southbank Polytechnic Distance Learning Centre.

CLIFFORD, C., CARNWELL, R. and HARKIN, L. (1997) *Research Methodology in Nursing and Healthcare*, Churchill Livingstone/Open Learning Foundation.

CLIFFORD, C. (1997) *Qualitative Research Methodology in Nursing and Healthcare*, Churchill Livingstone/Open Learning Foundation.

DALY, J. et al. (1992) *Researching Health Care: Designs, dilemmas, disciplines*, Routledge.

DENZIN, N.K. (1978) *The Research Act*, 2nd edition, McGraw-Hill, New York.

DINGWALL, R. and FOX, S. (1992) 'Health visitors' and social workers' perceptions of child-care problems', in Abbott, P. and Sapsford, R. (1992) *Research into Practice: A reader for nurses and the caring professions*, Open University Press.

GREENE, J. (1994) 'Qualitative programme evaluation – Practice and promise', in Denzin, N.K. and Lincoln, Y.S. (1994) *Handbook of Qualitative Research*, Sage.

GUBA, E.G. and LINCOLN, Y.S. (1989) *Fourth Generation Evaluation*, Sage.

GUBA, E.G. and LINCOLN, Y.S. (1994) 'Competing paradigms in qualitative research', in Denzin, N.K. and Lincoln, Y.S. (1994) *Handbook of Qualitative Research*, Sage.

HAILEY, D. (1992) 'The perspective of the policy maker on health care research and evaluation', in Daly, J., McDonald, I. and Willis, E. (Eds) *Researching Health Care: Designs, dilemmas, disciplines*, Routledge.

HALL, D. (1991) *Health for all Children*, Oxford Medical Publications.

HALVORSON, H.W., PIKE, D.K., REED, F.M., MCCLATCHEY, M.W. and GOSSELINK, C.A. (1993) 'Using qualitative methods to evaluate health service delivery in three rural Colorado communities', *Evaluation and the Health Professions*, Vol. **16**. No. 4.

JICK, T.D. (1979) 'Mixing Qualitative and Quantitative Methods: Triangulation in action', *Administrative Science Quarterly*, December 1979, Vol. **24**.

JONES ELWYN, G. and STOTT, N. (1994) 'Avoidable referrals? Analysis of 170 consecutive referrals to secondary care', *British Medical Journal*, Vol. **30**.

JUDD, C.M. (1987) 'Combining process and outcome evaluation', in Mark, M.M. and Shotland, R.L. (Eds) *Multiple methods in Programme Evaluation*, Jossey-Bass, San Francisco.

KEEBLE, S. (1995) *Experimental Research 1*, Healthcare Active Learning Series, Churchill Livingstone/Open Learning Foundation.

KENT, J. (1995) 'Evaluating pre-registration midwifery education', *Nursing Times*, Vol. **91**. No 24.

LEININGER, M. (1994) 'Evaluation criteria and critique of qualitative research studies', in Morse, J. (1994) *Critical Issues in Qualitative Research*, Sage.

MILES, M.B. and HUBERMAN, A.M. (1994) *Qualitative Data Analysis – An Expanded Sourcebook,* Second edition, Sage.

MILLS, C. (1995) 'Evaluation of primary nursing in a nursing development unit', *Nursing Times*, Vol. **91**. No. 39.

MULLEN, P.D. and IVERSON, D.C. (1986) 'Qualitative methods', in Green, I.W. and Lewis, F.M. (Eds) *Measurement and Evaluation in Health Education and Health Promotion*, Mayfield, Palo Alto.

ORR, J. (1992) 'Working with women's health groups: The community health movement', in Abbott, P. and Sapsford, R. (1992) *Research into Practice: A reader for nurses and the caring professions*, Open University Press.

PATTON, M.Q. (1986) *Utilisation-focused Evaluation*, Beverley Hills, Sage.

PATTON, M.Q. (1987) *How to Use Qualitative Methods in Evaluation*, Sage.

PHILLIPS, C., PALFREY, C. and THOMAS, P. (1994) *Evaluating Health and Social Care*, Macmillan.

POLIT, D.F. and HUNGLER, B.P. (1987) *Nursing Research: Principles and methods*, Third Edition, Lippincott, Philadelphia.

POPHAM, W.J. (1993) 'A strategy to encourage the evaluation of health education programmes', *Evaluation and the Health Professions*, Vol. **16**. No. 4.

REDFERN, S. J. and NORMAN, I. J. (1994) 'Validity through triangulation', *Nurse Researcher*, Vol. **2**. No 2. December.

REICHARDT, C.S. and COOK, T.T. (Eds.) (1979) *Qualitative and Quantitative Methods*, Sage.

SCRIVEN, M. (1967) 'The methodology of evaluation', AERA Monograph Series, in *Curriculum Evaluation*, **1**.

SCRIVEN, M. (1973) 'Goal-free evaluation', in House, E.R. (Ed) *School Evaluation: The politics and process*, McCutchan, Berkeley.

STAKE, R.E. (1978) 'The case study method in social enquiry', *Educational Researcher*, **71**. 1.

STAKE, R.E. (1991) Retrospective on 'The countenance of educational evaluation', in McLaughlin, M.W. and Phillips, D.C. (Eds) *Evaluation and Education: A quarter century*, University of Chicago Press, Chicago.

STECHER, B. M. and DAVIS, W. A. (1987) *How to Focus an Evaluation*, Sage.

SWANSON, J. M. and CHAPMAN, L. (1994) 'Inside the Black Box: Theoretical and methodological issues in conducting evaluation research using a qualitative approach', in Morse, J. (1994) *Critical Issues in Qualitative Research*, Sage.

THORPE, M. (1988) *Evaluating Open and Distance Learning*, Longman Open Learning.

WOODWARD, C.A. (1992) 'Broadening the scope of evaluation: Why and how', in Daly, J., McDonald, I. and Willis, E. (Eds) *Researching Health Care: Designs, dilemmas, disciplines*, Routledge.

GLOSSARY

Critical research –

A research approach in which the researcher gets involved with participants in order to enable and empower them to instigate social and political change.

Evaluation research –

An approach to research which aims to establish the value of a programme or service.

Exploratory research –

An approach in which the researcher explores the field of research in order to seek the opinions and feelings of the participants.

External validity –

The degree to which research results are generalisable to populations and samples other than those studied by the researcher.

Hypothesis –

A statement of the predicted relationship between two or more variables.

Hypothesis tail –

The number of outcomes identified within a hypothesis. Either one or two.

Inductive reasoning –

A process of reasoning from specific observations to general rules, so that knowledge is brought into view for the first time.

Interrogation –

A statement in question form which seeks to identify a gap in knowledge.

Level of significance –

The probability that an observed relationship between variables occurred by chance. A probability (p value) of 0.05 is normally acceptable, indicating that there is a five per cent chance that the observed relationship between variables was a chance occurrence rather than due to the manipulation of the variables by the researcher.

Likert scale –

An attitude scale which comprises a list of positively and negatively worded statements with which respondents are asked to indicate their strength of agreement or disagreement.

Nominal data –

The simplest level of measurement, in which dichotomous data are categorised into two groupings such as male/female, yes/no, pass/fail.

Non-probability sampling –

A type of sampling strategy in which there is no assurance that each member of the population has an equal chance of being selected.

Null hypothesis –

An hypothesis that states that there is no relationship between the variables defined in the experimental hypothesis.

Parametric test –

A test to establish the parameters of a population, usually based on the mean of a sample.

Positivism –

An approach to research which relies on the search for objective truth through quantitative measurements such as surveys and tightly controlled experiments.

Probability sampling –

A type of sampling strategy that assures each member of a population has an equal chance of being selected.

Quasi-experimental research –

a type of research in which the researcher manipulates the independent variable and exerts control over the study, but is unable to randomly allocate the subjects to experimental and control groups.

Sampling frame –

A list of all the elements (people) in the population from which the sample will be drawn for the research.

Stakeholder –

A term frequently used in evaluative research which refers to all the people who may have a stake in the service or programme to be evaluated. Stakeholders may include clients, staff, decision-makers and purchasers.

Test-retest reliability –

A method of assessing the reliability of a research instrument by distributing it to the same sample on different occasions and comparing the results. A high correlation between the sets of results indicates that the instrument is reliable in measuring the variables under consideration.

Time sampling –

A method of sampling used in observation research in which data are collected at regular intervals, such as every ten minutes, every hour or once a day.

Variable –

A characteristic of a person or object which takes on particular relevance depending on the research. For example, IQ might be a relevant variable for some research, whilst age, gender or weight might be relevant variables in other research.